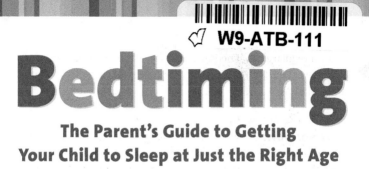

Bedtiming

The Parent's Guide to Getting Your Child to Sleep at Just the Right Age

Because sleep training is challenging and difficult, your child should be at his or her best when you begin. This handy reference guide sets out which ages and stages are problematic for getting your child to sleep and those that make it relatively easy. For more detail on these developmental windows, you can refer to the chart on pages 130 to 131 and the information in Chapter 4. Remember, the likelihood that your child will easily learn to sleep on his or her own has less to do with the precise technique you choose than with *when* you try to apply it.

0 TO 2½ MONTHS

WHY NOT NOW? There is too much going on. Your baby's body needs time to develop and stabilize its own cycles. Because of that, it may be difficult or impossible to establish desirable sleep habits before sleeping at night becomes routine.

WHAT YOU CAN DO INSTEAD: Whatever gets you through the night. Rocking, bouncing, cuddling and gliding are all great options. Anything you do, you can undo with proper sleep training at a later stage of development.

2½ TO 4 MONTHS

WHY NOW? This is a period of relative stability and resilience. There is no good reason not to try sleep training at this age if your intuition says "go!" and your baby responds favorably. Some parents, however, feel that this age is just too early to start sleep training, so trust your instincts.

WHAT YOU SHOULD KNOW: Young babies have a hard time recovering from intense distress, and past a certain threshold (about 5 to 10 minutes) they may continue to cry until exhaustion sets in. This may be a signal that now is not the right time. If intense distress continues to be a regular part of bedtime after a week, it can be another sign that now isn't the right time. If that's the case, we suggest you wait for the next window.

✘ 4 TO 5½ MONTHS

WHY NOT NOW? As your baby learns new interpersonal skills—skills that call for expected responses from you and lead to a stronger bond between you—it's better not to disturb them until they've really begun to solidify. Essentially, sleep training at this age can cause frustration and confusion because your baby needs you to be her playmate, not her disciplinarian.

WHAT YOU CAN DO INSTEAD: Avoid compounding this period of often stressful growth with the added stress of sleep training—both for you and your baby. Continue to establish predictable and consistent bedtime routines, but don't push anything that doesn't feel right.

✔ 5½ TO 7½ MONTHS (AN IDEAL TIME)

WHY NOW? Babies are engaged with the world of objects around them (more than they are with people) and show almost no signs of separation distress. This combination creates one of the best times for sleep training. Sleep train any earlier and your baby is less stable. Sleep train any later and your baby will feel the pangs of separation distress to at least some degree.

WHAT YOU SHOULD KNOW: Your baby will probably start to grow out of swaddling at this point, if that's a technique you've been using. Consider how you might orchestrate sleep training with moving away from swaddling so that your baby doesn't have to deal with the stress of both at once.

To really get a full night's sleep, you'll need to eliminate night feeding. Try gradually reorganizing your baby's feeding schedule so that he consumes most of his nourishment during the day.

Nighttime noise may be a bigger problem than ever before as your baby becomes more alert to what's going on around him. Try running a fan for white noise.

✘ 8 TO 11 MONTHS (ONE OF THE WORST TIMES)

WHY NOT NOW? Separation now means something to your baby—that you're not responding to his attempts to bring you back—which can be upsetting and traumatic for your baby and destructive to your attempts at sleep training.

WHAT YOU CAN DO INSTEAD: Continue to be consistent in your bedtime routines but be responsive to your baby's needs. This stage will pass!

✔ 12 TO 16 MONTHS

WHY NOW? This is another emotionally stable period where your baby is as focused on the world around her as she is on you. The challenges at this stage will involve your now-toddler's energetic spirit and intelligence. If your child still isn't sleeping through the night, this may be your last chance for an efficient and fully satisfactory sleep-training experience, so stick with it!

WHAT YOU SHOULD KNOW: Play—not sleep—is number one on your baby's list of priorities. You'll need to balance loving attention and concern with a firm determination to avoid the tricks and traps your innovative toddler will use to avoid bedtime.

✘ 17 TO 21 MONTHS

WHY NOT NOW? Sleep training at this age is bound to be hampered by two interlocking issues: your toddler's fear of separation and his determination to hold his own in conflict situations.

WHAT YOU CAN DO INSTEAD: Wait it out. The small amount of sleep you might gain isn't worth the battle. Stay consistent in bedtime routines, but be gentle on yourself and on your emerging Terrible Two.

✔ 22 TO 27 MONTHS

WHY NOW? Even if you've done successful sleep training before this stage, some of it has probably come undone in the last few months. But now your child is more calm, more stable, and more secure than she was just recently.

WHAT YOU SHOULD KNOW: Introduce sleep training a little differently by involving rules and goals, because that's what 2-year-olds understand best. Sleep training will be trickier at this stage than at any previous one, because your toddler has a much more finely tuned ability to manipulate situations to get what he wants. Make sure that fun bedtime routines involving stories, songs and cuddly stuffed animals make the rewards of good sleep habits obvious to him.

✗ 28 MONTHS TO 3 YEARS

WHY NOT NOW? A tricky combination of a capacity for intense jealousy and a willingness to push boundaries makes for a determined yet irrational little girl or boy. By this age, though, children's development becomes quite individual, so follow your instincts as to what is right for your child.

WHAT YOU CAN DO INSTEAD: Give sleep training a pass for several months if your child is prone to jealousy, if he is on the defiant end of the spectrum, or if he tends to wage battles whenever rules and regulations are not carved in stone. If your child has an easier disposition, if he already seems comfortable and relaxed about his role in the family, it might not be necessary to wait any longer. In either case, consistency is key.

✔ 3 TO 3½ YEARS

WHY NOW? This is the last window of opportunity to initiate or repair sleeping habits with ease. Your child is motivated to be a valued member of the family, and you can use that concern to your advantage.

WHAT YOU SHOULD KNOW: Stuffed animals or other cuddly items are a key tool for bedtime comfort, as are well-established family routines for bedtime.

✗ 3½ TO 4 YEARS

WHY NOT NOW? Feelings of shame can be debilitating for some children starting around 3½ years of age; sleep training should be avoided for these sensitive kids. While they are lying in bed alone, children have plenty of time to ruminate on what their parents might be thinking about them. And if those thoughts include images of rejection, disapproval, or even abandonment, then they may lead to habitual worries that will eventually crystallize into long-lasting insecurities.

WHAT YOU CAN DO INSTEAD: Reassure your child that sleeping alone isn't about being excluded from anything, but more about being a big girl or boy. This will lead to a growing sense of self-esteem.

Keep in mind that many factors can disrupt hard-won sleep skills, and you may find yourself teaching these skills again, in an entirely different developmental window. So even if you've used this book once to identify the best age to sleep train, you may want to keep your copy handy, in case a sleep setback requires you to find another optimal window for retraining your child.

Bedtiming

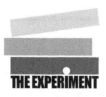

THE EXPERIMENT

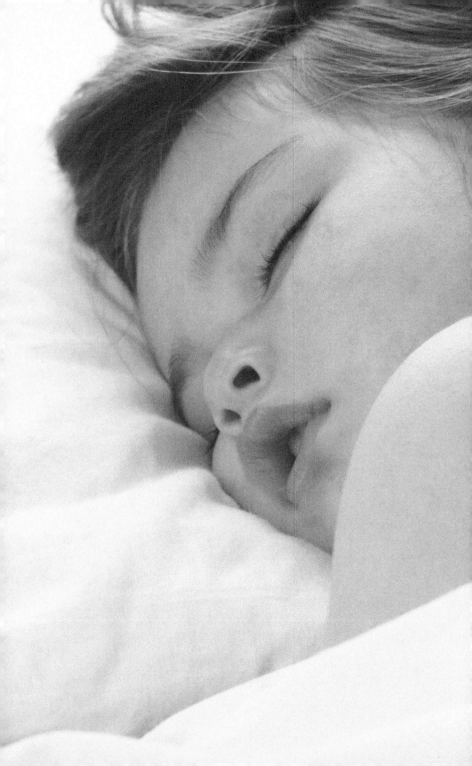

Bedtiming

The Parent's Guide to Getting Your Child to Sleep
at Just the Right Age

Marc D. Lewis, PhD
Isabela Granic, PhD

THE EXPERIMENT
NEW YORK

The Experiment, LLC
220 East 23rd Street, Suite 301
New York, NY 10010-4674
www.theexperimentpublishing.com

First U.S. edition published by arrangement with HarperCollins Canada Ltd.

Photo credits:
Pages ii–iii, 14: Ekaterina Monakhova; page viii: Rosemarie Gearhart; pages 48, 210: Gloria-Leigh Logan; page 126: Evelin Elmest/all iStockphoto; page 184: Monkey Business Images/Dreamstime

Library of Congress Control Number: 2009937034
ISBN 978-1-61519-015-7

Cover design by Alison Forner
Cover photograph © OJO Images/SuperStock
Author photograph by Jennifer Pearson Photography
Design by Sharon Kish

Manufactured in the United States of America
First printing January 2010
10 9 8 7 6

Contents

1   **Timing Is Everything**   **1**

2   **How Your Child Thinks**
    Cognitive Development in the First 4 Years   **15**

3   **How Your Child Feels**
    Emotional Development in the First 4 Years   **49**

4   **Windows of Opportunity**
    When to Sleep Train and When to Wait   **127**

5   **The Pros and Cons of**
    Popular Sleep-Training Methods   **185**

6   **Sleep Setbacks and How to Handle Them**   **211**

    Acknowledgments   **222**
    Bibliography   **224**
    Index   **226**

1

Timing Is Everything

SLEEP DOESN'T SEEM LIKE SUCH A BIG DEAL until you begin to go without it. That's why, out of all the complaints, worries, stresses, and strains we hear about from parents of babies and toddlers, sleep deprivation is by far the most frequent and often the most troublesome. Of course this is common knowledge. Tell your coworkers that you have a young baby at home, and the first thing you'll hear back is "Good luck sleeping!" Your own parents, having been through the ordeal with you and your siblings, will regard you with a mix of sympathy and vindication: So *now* you know what it's like. They might be there to help for the first few weeks, waking up with you every 3 hours to feed, taking on a bottle-feeding of their own, standing watch while you nap during the day, desperately trying to catch up. But inevitably, you're on your own. In a vast majority of families in North America, it's the parents—and most often the mother—who can't get enough sleep for the first few months, or even years, of the child's life. And inadequate sleep has many costs.

You are confronting one of the most challenging tasks of your life: raising an infant or toddler. There is no rule book telling you exactly what to do and when to do it, what works and what doesn't, no matter how persistently you browse the parenting section of your bookstore. You have to use your intuition, your common sense, and your problem-solving abilities, at peak efficiency, many times throughout the day. And this is all the more true if you have other major demands on your time—other children to raise, a husband (or wife) to put through school, or work outside the home to attend to. Not only your ability to think clearly but also your ability to maintain emotional equilibrium is of utmost importance. You can't afford to get into a frustrated rage, or a depression, or a state of persistent irritation. You can't afford to blow up at your husband, your other children, or your boss. And you certainly can't afford to become resentful of this baby who, as cute and delightful as she may be, is the source of your sleeplessness. Mental acuity and emotional stability are absolutely essential to the parent of a young child.

And yet you can hardly see straight! You slept for 5 hours last night. Well, that's stretching it. You actually slept for 1½ hours on average during each of three periods between 10 p.m. and 7 a.m. Because the baby was crying. The baby was hungry. The baby needed changing. The baby needed to be rocked. Nobody knows what the baby needed, but he sure was hollering until you picked him up. Or, your toddler, who never really did sleep very well, crawled into bed with you eight times after he was supposedly asleep, and each time you had to wake up and cuddle him and then take him back to his bed, or nurse him, or play with him. Or you've been co-sleeping with your baby blissfully for months, but now he's realized that bedtime is really a great playtime, and so no one in the family is getting any sleep. What's worse, the nearly 5 hours of sleep you'd like to think you logged turns out to include only 2 hours of solid sleep because, come to think of it, you were really only half asleep for a few of those hours, lying there drifting in and out of dreams, in a state of, let's face it: dread. Just waiting for the next bout of screaming, the next scratch at the door, the next cry of "Mommy!" from down the hall. It's no wonder you can hardly see straight. Your capacity to reason has dwindled to the most basic computations: *got to warm up the food, got to chop it first, last jar of fruit, put it on the list.* Your long-term memory is a joke. Did you decide to let him cry it out at nap time, or was that a dream? Or were you talking about next month? Was it the carrots he spit all over you in a show of primal disgust, or was that the sweet potato? And your emotions are all over the map. You kept it together splendidly when the cat knocked over both bottles of milk, even though the baby was screaming in apparent agony for a full 15 minutes. Yet you blew up at the cable guy because nobody told you about the extra fee for the second outlet. And you and your husband haven't really been on the best of terms since that argument, yesterday morning, about when to start your child in a playgroup. In fact you've barely looked at each other. Sometimes it's safer that way.

You Snooze or You Lose

If you're like most parents, you have felt pangs of guilt because of your desire to *sleep train* your baby. Maybe even the term gives you the creeps, just a little. Training sounds like something you do with a pet, after all. But more to the point, putting your own sleep needs (desperate as they may be) before your baby's sense of emotional security seems like the epitome of poor parenting. Mothers in particular are often given the message by the media, friends, and family (including fellow mothers, unfortunately) that their first and only priority should be their child's happiness. Parents' own health and well-being should be considered secondary, if at all.

We want to dispel this dangerous myth right away. Parents who are considering sleep training their babies for reasons beyond the well-being of their child (gasp!) not only are perfectly normal but also are *doing the right thing.* A sleep-deprived family is an unhappy, unhealthy one. And this unhealthy state of affairs has massive implications for parenting and the child's long-term well-being. Here are just a few facts we've compiled about the necessity of sleep. The significance of this sleep research for improving parents' lives as well as their actual parenting ability seems crystal clear.

- A new baby typically deprives parents of 400 to 750 hours of sleep in the first year.
- Being awake for 17 hours straight leads to the same kind of impairment as a blood alcohol level of .05 percent (you could be arrested for driving at that level).
- Fatigue is involved in approximately one in six fatal road accidents.
- Sleep deprivation affects both long- and short-term memory.
- High-level problem-solving skills are most impaired by lack of sleep (this would include figuring out the best way to help your child sleep better, making the right choices for

child care, and figuring out how to mix the formula, avoid allergens, give the right dose of reflux medication, and so on).

- Prolonged sleep deprivation has been linked repeatedly to depression (and many studies have shown that untreated maternal depression can have serious long-term effects on child adjustment).
- Some studies have shown that women need an hour more sleep than men per night; not getting this extra sleep may be one reason why women are far more susceptible to depression than men.

> You can't be the effective
> parent you want to be
> if you're exhausted.

In short, your sleep is as important as your baby's. You just can't be the parent you want to be if you're exhausted, crabby, and irrational. And when parents don't get enough sleep at night, the household starts to fall apart. Quite literally, your parenting, your work, and oftentimes the quality of your marriage will start to unravel if you don't get enough sleep to feel and function normally. Too many nighttime wakings and inadequate napping schedules are unhealthy for the young child too. Babies, toddlers, and older children need their sleep, or else they are likely to be fussy. Their moods in turn affect your mood. It's harder to be patient and sympathetic to a kid who is irritable and whiny. Then your shortened fuse—a result of your fatigue—may lead to further behavioral and emotional difficulties for your child, all of which gives rise to a vicious cycle of irritability, discontent, sleep problems, and ongoing fatigue. The sleep-deprived child also finds it more difficult to pay attention for any stretch of time, she's less likely to learn quickly and remember what she's learned, and these sleep-related problems develop into habits, or learning styles, that can persist into adolescence and adulthood.

This is how one mother sums up the time before she decided to sleep train.

ANNE'S STORY
Hitting the Wall

It took 9 months of Freeda getting up at least 10 times per night before I finally broke down. A lifelong history of insomnia gives you an increased tolerance of sleep deprivation, which held me in good stead under the circumstances. But still. There was the Wall, and I ran smack-dab into it, with enough force that it left a nice brick pattern in my forehead.

The Wall went something like this: Every time Freeda woke me up at night, I swore. I muttered angry nothings under my breath. Every day, if Freeda wouldn't nap (and I wasn't even trying the crib; it was the BabyBjörn carrier for every nap), I cried. I cried when she woke up. I cranked at my husband constantly. I was miserable in both senses of the word: I felt miserable, and I was miserable to be with. And one day, when I found myself shouting at my precious, so-beloved baby to just "SLEEP, GODDAMNIT—WOULD IT KILL YOU TO SLEEP?" there it was. A nice brick wall.

On that wall was a sign: "Do you really think this constant anger and exhaustion benefits your attachment to your baby? What's better—a few nights or weeks of crying from sleep training and a happy, rested mommy forever, or a quick and bitter response at night, every night, and a mommy who is muttering death threats? Think, woman, *think*."

So I bought a book on sleep training. Actually, I bought several. I bought every book in the bookstore and even borrowed a few from the library. I read them all. I selected from each author the parts of their approaches that seemed to suit my wee girl. And while my husband was away on business, I put them into effect.

Who Needs Another Book on Sleep Training?

To rectify young children's sleep problems, a number of books have come out over the past 20 years or so addressing the theme of "sleep training." Sleep training is any technique for teaching your child to sleep through the night as much as possible and nap regularly and sufficiently through the day. Our definition of sleep training also includes transitioning children from the family bed to their own cribs or beds and teaching them to sleep alone in their own rooms.

There are quite a few popular sleep-training books. Many of these offer sound, practical advice on how to teach, train, tempt, cajole, or coerce your baby, toddler, or preschooler to sleep when you want him to sleep. Some of them also suggest changes in household strategies or routines, like nap schedules, to help your child be bright and happy during the day and sleep soundly at night. And some focus on broader issues, like the pros and cons of a family bed, as well as other household patterns likely to have an impact on children's sleep problems. These books also offer excellent problem-solving tips on how to overcome the challenges that make particular children "difficult" when it comes to sleeping. We find that sleep-training books vary widely on the type of interventions they recommend. At one extreme are those that suggest little to no intervention. They advocate letting children cry, sometimes for more than an hour, as they "teach themselves" to fall asleep. At the other extreme are techniques that are supposed to avoid letting the child cry while he is learning to fall asleep and sleep through the night. We strongly believe that almost all of these sleep-training techniques are valuable in some way and that it is up to the parents to choose the one that best matches their parenting style and philosophy, their cultural background, their child's temperament, family structure, and so on.

However, each and every sleep training book ignores one critical issue: the question of *when* (at what age) to apply the technique it offers. Some books provide vague guidelines, or comment briefly on a single period that may or may not be ideal. Yet no one has set out a timetable of developmental periods during which you are most likely to be successful at sleep training. And no one has attempted to use scientific knowledge about child development to devise such a schedule. We find this remarkable. With all the good advice out there on what to do and how to do it, parents still need a well-reasoned guide to the periods of development during which sleep training is likely to work smoothly in contrast to those most likely to be difficult, to be emotionally stressful for the child and parent, or to fail entirely.

Knowing *when* to sleep train is more important than knowing *how*.

The success of sleep training is highly dependent on when you attempt it. In fact, the *when* of sleep training is more important than the *how*. There are certain ages at which babies and toddlers are ready to learn to fall asleep easily and stay asleep through most if not all of the night. There are other ages at which, no matter what method you choose, your baby or toddler seems determined to resist your efforts, leading to an escalation in the crying, screaming, stress, and heartache that you badly wanted to avoid. One parent's story says it all.

KAREN'S STORY
Bye-Bye Rock-a-Bye

Okay, I will admit I have always rocked my boy to sleep. Of course, now I am paying dearly for it! He's almost 9 months old and cannot go to sleep on his own. I want to let him cry it out, but he spits up a lot. . . . I can't go in while he's crying, because that will just make him more hysterical. He also gets super clingy the day after I try to get him to cry himself to sleep. When I do it, he never lets me put him down the next day!

The absence of knowledge about developmental timing is by far the biggest factor sabotaging sleep training. And this is a real tragedy for many families. The parents try sleep training once or twice, at precisely the wrong ages, and encounter such negative results that they never try again. These are the parents who have learned to live with 4 to 5 hours of sleep per night. They are not happy campers—they have dark bags under their eyes—but they've never figured out where they went wrong.

Reading this book will ensure that as parents of young children you no longer have to join the ranks of the walking dead. We want to give you the knowledge you need to apply your preferred method of sleep training—whatever it is—in the right developmental periods. Some people assume that sleep training is best accomplished early in development, when babies are still pliable and before they develop entrenched habits. This is the *earlier-is-better* school of thought. Other people assume that sleep training works better when children are older, once they have developed a secure bond with their parents and feel safe and confident in the family and in the world at large. This is the *later-is-better* school of thought. We strongly believe that both of these assumptions are wrong. In fact, they fly in the face of contemporary theory and research in developmental psychology.

Development does not look like a smooth ramp that goes either up or down, continuously, from birth to some later age. Rather, development is a sequence of stages, or phases, or periods, each with its own characteristics, its own strengths and weaknesses, its own vulnerabilities and resiliencies. In several of his books, developmental psychologist Jerome Kagan, at Harvard

University, emphasizes how thoroughly children differ from one stage to the next—so much so that they seem more similar to other children in the same stage than to their previous selves! This stage-by-stage variation is the basis of our approach in this book. During some periods of development, young children are not particularly vulnerable to separations from parents or to the frustration of having their demands go unmet. These are ideal periods in which to commence and to succeed at sleep training. During other periods, children are highly attuned to their parents' whereabouts, especially to sudden separations, to their parents' responses to their demands, to competition with other family members, and to changes of any kind in family rituals. These are the wrong times to embark on sleep training, because it will usually fail or else catch on finally after long hours of crying. Luckily, these developmental periods tend to correspond to highly predictable age ranges, at least within a given society. This allows us to attach age estimates to each developmental stage, estimates that turn out to be remarkably precise and reliable.

The particular qualities, opportunities, and challenges of each developmental stage can be understood only by examining the cognitive capabilities and emotional issues characteristic of that stage. And because cognitive capacities and emotional issues change—rapidly and sometimes counterintuitively, forming an intricate and convoluted patchwork—common sense is a poor yardstick for assessing them. That's why this book is based on a solid body of theory and research that has been accumulating in developmental psychology over the last four decades. Both authors are developmental psychologists. Isabel is a research scientist at the Hospital for Sick Children and Marc is a professor at the University of Toronto. We know the literature on child development and we have published several dozen articles in scientific journals contributing to that literature. Marc is also a direct descendant (in the academic sense) of Jean Piaget, the preeminent stage theorist of the 20th century: his mentor's mentor's mentor was Piaget. And we are parents ourselves. Our twin boys are 2 years old at the time of writing. We know how difficult parenting can be, despite its many rewards, and how the most commonplace routines can go amiss if the details are slightly off. We think that these two sources of knowledge—the theoretical and the practical—help us to understand the big picture as well as the nuts and bolts when it comes to the challenge of shaping your child's sleep habits. And so we hope that the schedule of ages and stages provided in this book will help you where you need it most, not to replace but to complement the techniques you may already be trying or plan to try. We want to make those methods as effective and painless as possible.

How to Use This Book

If you have enough time to sit down and read for an hour or two per day, and you're not excessively fatigued right now, we suggest you read this book from start to finish. The structure of the book is designed to lead you smoothly from foundational principles, through a detailed examination of age-specific emotional issues, to a concrete road map of ages and stages most likely and least likely to lend themselves to sleep training, and finally to the implications of different temperaments and sleep-training methods. However, if you're tired, stressed, perhaps even feeling desperate, if you haven't had a good night's sleep for as long as you can remember, if getting your child to sleep is really all you can think about at the moment, then we suggest you jump immediately to Chapter 4. This chapter identifies the stages of development least appropriate for sleep training and those most likely to lead to success without emotional trauma. It also provides a comprehensive table where these periods are displayed, along with their probable age boundaries and a summary version of the psychological issues underlying them. In fact, this table (Figure 3, pages 130 to 131) is where to look first if you have only a minute or two between one emergency and the next. Then, as you start to get better rested, or more interested in the reasons behind the developmental sequence of your child's behavior, or both, you can return to the earlier chapters at your—dare we say?—leisure. Once your child is sleeping soundly through the night and napping regularly during the day, you'll find that you're ready to think about a lot of things. In fact, thinking itself will seem like a marvelous new pastime, waiting to flower in your well-rested mind and body.

Meanwhile, happy reading, and be assured (soon, *rest* assured) that you are far from alone. Good sleep habits don't appear automatically in most children's lives. But with a little knowledge taken from developmental psychology, application of some principles and practices, and especially careful attention to developmental *timing*, those habits can easily be attained. And once your child's sleep problems are firmly in the past tense, life will be more relaxed and a lot more fun for everyone in the family.

2

How Your Child Thinks

Cognitive Development in the First 4 Years

PERHAPS THE MAIN BIOLOGICAL DIFFERENCE between humans and other animals is that our brains continue to develop for a very long time after birth. Our brains are not completely formed until sometime after the adolescent years. It is no coincidence that this long period of maturation is recognized by every culture as requiring care and support, only gradually giving way to the responsibilities of "adulthood." In fact, it is during this period that the growth and maturation of the brain is scaffolded by intense practices of care, socialization, and teaching, so that the finished product—the young adult—truly belongs to the culture and community in which she developed.

But the entire brain does not grow uniformly over the years of childhood. Most regions of the brain have already assumed their basic shape before birth. Much of the hardware and software responsible for sensation, arousal, physiological maintenance, coordinated action, and even, to some degree, emotion is already functioning effectively in young babies. However, the cerebral cortex changes massively, rewiring itself almost completely. The cortex is the light gray convoluted tissue that surrounds all other brain structures, made up of 10 to 20 billion cells densely connected with one another. It is the part of the brain we see, the part that looks familiar from medical documentaries and horror movies. And it is the part of the brain that we hold responsible for "thought," which includes planning, evaluation, memory organization, speech, perception, and direct action. It is also the part of the brain whose finely chiseled structure determines differences in personality and social disposition. We see this unique organization emerge—grow and consolidate—in child development. And sometimes, tragically, we see portions of it disintegrate when individuals suffer from a stroke or other brain damage.

The cortex is generally considered the highest level of brain evolution, and indeed our cortices are much larger, and have much, much greater surface area, than those of even our closest animal relatives. So, what does it mean to say that the cortex continues to take shape and get organized long after birth? One consequence of delayed cortical maturation is that thought, perception, planning, and action capabilities do not develop in the dark chamber of the womb. Rather, these capacities develop while the child is actively moving about, exploring and receiving feedback from the world at the same time. The developing cortex is being guided during all these processes by parents, siblings, and other (more experienced!) humans. In other words, the brain grows as it works, through social interaction, to make sense of an incredibly complex and changing world. In this way, brain development can never be seen as "just biological." Brain development is the result of a two-way communication between changes in the child's own body and changes in the social world—primarily the family: a communication that continuously filters, categorizes, and makes sense of all the child's experiences. And the family inevitably adjusts to the growing child, just as the growing child adjusts to the family.

> The developing brain is shaped by social interactions with caregivers and other important people in the child's life.

Experience feeds the brain with information about the world—and not just any world, but the world in which the infant, toddler, and eventually the child happens to live. It is a very specific world, depending on the number and layout of rooms in the house, the available toys, the hazards in the environment, siblings and their actions, the kinds of books on the bookshelf, the number of hours the TV is on, and parents' personalities, behavior, income, and education. Experience teaches the brain about a *relevant* world. At the same time, the brain has its own capacities. It is a biological organ, and it has limits. Some of these limits can be seen in real time—minutes and hours. For example, there is only so much one can read before becoming mentally "full," just as there is only so much we can eat before the stomach reaches its capacity. But other limits shown by the brain can be seen only in development, in the amount and kind of change that is achieved over several months or years. These limits include, most importantly, a speed limit on development. Brains cannot change instantly. They change at a certain rate. Like muscles, whose growth takes time no matter how much they are exercised, the brain's rate of change is constrained by its biological makeup, no matter how "enriched" the environment. In fact, the timetable of brain growth, its schedule of development, is largely independent of the specific features of the child's environment. This schedule depends, instead, on mechanisms of growth of various kinds of brain cells, processes by which brain cells become connected with one another, mechanisms for making neural transmission more efficient, and the ways those mechanisms interact with the social world. This "universal" timetable of growth is why parents and grandparents for centuries have been able to celebrate baby's first smile around 3 months, commiserate about their "clingy" 9-month-old, and laugh about the seemingly inevitable "Terrible Twos." Ask any experienced nanny in the park what to do with a toddler who refuses to eat anything but olives, and she'll say: "Wait until he's 4."

The Timetable of Cognitive Development

We suggest that the limits and constraints of cortical growth create a particular timetable for cognitive development. This timetable was well known—and in fact largely discovered—by Jean Piaget, a Swiss scholar and developmental thinker whose enormous impact on the study of child development stemmed from more than 60 years of research. (Piaget began his scientific work as a teenager and did not stop until his death in 1980, at the age of 84.) Indeed, a maturing brain in a more or less normal environment has a fairly expectable schedule of changes. These changes support eye contact with mother at 3 months, grabbing and sucking on toys at 5 to 6 months, searching for vanished objects at 9 months, and racing off to explore the world at 13 to 14 months. Most important, the schedule of cognitive development—changes in the thinking, perceiving, and planning part of the brain—can be viewed as the backbone of all other areas of development, including emotional and social development. The schedule of cognitive stages provides us with a timetable for emotional stages. And this emotional timetable is the key that determines how your child will respond to your attempts to teach him how to fall asleep easily at a given age. In the next chapter, we look at how cognitive developmental milestones translate to emotional milestones. Here, we map out the timetable of cognitive changes, partly because most parents find them fascinating on their own.

To provide the most up-to-date picture of the stages of cognitive development, we now go beyond Piaget to the "neo-Piagetian" theories that extend his insights. Piaget divided development into four major stages, each of which is further divided into substages. The major stages are often described as (1) sensorimotor, (2) preoperational, (3) concrete operational, and (4) formal operational. Virtually all of the important stage theories that followed Piaget have taken the same tack: they describe three or four major stages, each divided into three or four substages. One of the most influential of these theories was proposed by Robbie Case, a brilliant researcher at the University of Toronto who spanned the disciplines of developmental and educational psychology. For Case, the four major stages of childhood are labeled (1) sensorimotor (just like Piaget), (2) interrelational, (3) dimensional, and (4) vectorial, and these stages correspond quite closely, both in age and in quality, to Piaget's stages. Here we are interested in the first two stages of the lifespan: the sensorimotor stage extends from 4 to 18 months, and the interrelational stage extends from 18 months (1½ years) to about 5 years. These two stages contain three substages each, with the addition of a preliminary substage from birth to 4 months, altogether totaling seven substages from birth to 5 years.

But to make all this more digestible, we will simply chart the first seven substages (we'll call them stages) of the lifespan, labeling them according to the skills and capacities that arise within each. We will use Case's theory to explain how specific behaviors, capacities, and skills appear in the child's repertoire at predictable ages, based on the cognitive activities, or mental events, supported by the child's brain as it matures with experience over the early years of life. We will also use Case's age ranges to pinpoint the boundaries of each stage, as we have found them to be impressively accurate both through research and anecdotes shared by countless parents. You will no doubt recognize many of the features that emerge within each stage. (It's almost as if babies came equipped with an actual timetable!) But first, it is important to mention the engine that propels cognitive development and moves the developing child from one stage to the next.

The Engine of Cognitive Development: Working Memory

Robbie Case died just a few years ago, at age 56, and while still a very productive scholar. Many of those who learned from him, including the authors of this volume, continue to miss him and feel saddened by his loss. But like many famous psychologists, Case filled a place in an ongoing lineage, in particular, a lineage that comes straight from Piaget. Case's academic mentor was Juan Pascual-Leone, and Pascual-Leone's mentor was Piaget himself. Pascual-Leone's major contribution was to modernize Piaget's theory by introducing the concept of working memory and explaining how it could be responsible for stages of development. Working memory is the "buffer" that stores a certain number of pieces of information. It is very close to the idea of "short-term memory," and it functions like the RAM in your computer. Each piece of information can be thought of as a feature of a problem that needs to be solved. For example, your working memory is now filled up with the subject and predicate of this sentence, the meaning of the previous sentence, the overall thrust of this paragraph, and perhaps even your awareness of reading these words and making sense of them (now that we have drawn your attention to this fact). Pascual-Leone discovered that children's working memory increases with age, in an orderly fashion, and that these increases underlie their ability to think more elaborate thoughts and to plan more elaborate strategies.

Working memory is similar to short-term memory: it's the "buffer" that stores a certain amount of information in the moment.

Current theory and data suggest that increases in working memory reflect increased speed of information processing, and this speeding up results from the development of the frontal cortex (the front third of the cortex) and the filling in of its connections with other parts of the cortex. As it matures, the frontal cortex processes information more quickly and efficiently, allowing it to compile more complex images of the world and more complex strategies for acting on the world. In turn, these advances shift the child from one developmental stage to the next. In a sense, each stage represents a more sophisticated solution to a problem—a solution that is more integrated, more comprehensive, more abstract, and more powerful than the one before. Problem solving relies on the assembly of several pieces of information in working memory, and faster information processing allows children to hold more information in working memory at the same time.

Case's major contribution to the field was to describe stages of cognitive development in detail, demonstrate in some clever experiments their working memory requirements, and investigate the development of knowledge in a variety of domains (e.g., social reasoning, numerical reasoning, spatial reasoning). In essence, Case showed how a developing child can think, plan, and perceive in more and more powerful ways, in every area of mental activity, and how that progression falls naturally into a series of stages or periods, each of which has a character all its own.

For example, a 6-month-old baby is perfectly capable of grabbing a toy or other object in order to explore it close up (often by putting it in her mouth). This deed requires the coordination of two simple cognitions—sending the hand over to the location of the toy and then closing the hand around the toy to grasp it. However, a 9-month-old infant can do something much more sophisticated: he can squawk while looking at Dad with the expectation that he will pick up a fallen toy and hand it over! This improvement is roughly as momentous as building a bridge to cross a river rather than trying to jump it. Yet, this major advance depends on only one thing: putting together four pieces (or two pairs) of information (in working memory) rather than just two. Instead of just coordinating the reach command with the grasp command, the child can now coordinate the object's graspability, his own inability to reach far enough to grasp it, the image of his father's reach for the object, and his directed vocalization (with its expected impact on his father). This advance in information processing propels the infant from one stage of development to another, more sophisticated stage. Similar kinds of advances move the child from one stage to the next across the months and years of cognitive development. Figure 1 on pages 26 to 27 shows the schedule of these stages over the first 5 years of life.

Let's examine the stages of early cognitive development in some detail. The names of the stages are explained in the following passages, but for now the age range and content of each stage will be visible at a glance in Figure 1. The age ranges listed here should apply to most average children growing up in more or less average environments. But some variation in timing is to be expected, and variation is not meant in any way to be taken as a bad thing. For example, some babies are born prematurely and so their timing should correspond more to their "adjusted" age (to the expected due date rather than the actual date of their birth). Our twins, for instance, were born about a month before their due date and tended to hit the stage transitions about a month later than their same-age peers, at least in infancy.

Stage 1
Orienting: 0 to 4 months

Prior to 4 or 4½ months, babies simply can't do much with their arms and hands, and they can't move their hands to places where their eyes tell them they will find interesting things to hold. They can gaze at interesting objects continuously. They orient to them, if objects are already in their field of vision, and even track them as they move around. That's how they follow their parents with their gaze, becoming familiar with the changes in the size and shape of images—changes that mean they are coming closer or moving farther away. By 3 or 4 months, babies can track more complex movements, such as those of a mobile, and they take delight in the continuous changes of shape for which mobiles are famous. And beyond the realm of vision, there are things babies can do with their hands: they can hold on to a rattle, grasping it with their palm and fingers and feeling its texture. They can even put their hands into their mouths—with luck. But they can't coordinate their gaze with their manual actions. So the grasping they do is not guided by the visual system. And their gaze at objects rarely leads to reaching or grasping. Infants of this age are stuck in the first stage of cognitive development, when their capabilities are best characterized by what they *can't* do. According to Case, their limitations stem from their inability to coordinate two motor commands, or a perceptual (e.g., visual) image with a motor command, within their working memories. This inability to coordinate mental operations makes young infants unable to launch a two-part action, or an action intended to produce an effect. So all they can do is to continue more or less whatever they're already doing. If they're lucky enough to catch sight of a moving mobile, they can keep on gazing at it for some time. What they can't do is to purposely find it once it's out of sight.

A good way to get a handle on the stages of cognitive development is to describe the transitions from one to the next. Both authors studied some of these transitions in the Department of Human Development and Applied Psychology at the University of Toronto, under the tutelage of Robbie Case. Other descriptions come from other colleagues and students of Case. The transition from Stage 1 to 2 is quite dramatic. From relatively passive creatures, who do little with their hands or reach jerkily in the general direction of something appealing, babies evolve into goal-directed beings, intent on getting an expected reaction to their pushes and pulls, their reaches, their shifts in gaze direction, and above all the squawks and coos they direct at those hulking adults who are always hanging around. Within just a few weeks' time, they change from little blobs, painstakingly learning to get their hands, arms, and gaze to cooperate with their wishes into determined engines of intention, who grab for a particular purple elephant because that's what they want to explore. In Stage 1, the problems they can solve are very simple

Figure 1. Stages of Cognitive Development Over the First Five Years of Life

Approx. Age	Cognitive Stage	Cognitive Capacities
0–4 months	Stage 1 Orienting	Babies engage with their environment through simple actions or sensory attunement. Infants can • focus attention on one object at a time • perform unitary actions such as reaching or grasping • orient to interesting or exciting events • maintain attention However, they cannot coordinate reaching and grasping or switch their attention elsewhere.
4–8 months	Stage 2 Actions & Outcomes	Infants undergo a major shift to coordinated cognition, allowing for the dawning of intelligence. Infants can • coordinate reaching and grasping • coordinate gazing and reaching • engage in intentional acts • reach for objects to explore or put in mouth • expect actions (such as banging or shouting) to produce specific effects on objects or people
8–12 months	Stage 3 Point & Click	Double coordination takes hold as children "click" to the social world at last. Infants can • coordinate intentional acts with vocalizations or gestures aimed at other people • follow another's gaze • follow pointing and point to objects for others to see • interpret cues • recruit other people to obtain something • retrieve hidden objects from behind barriers

12–18 months	Stage 4 Honing Skills	Practice of double coordination allows for more complex problem solving, games, and social rituals. Infants can • place objects in containers and then remove them • place objects in matching locations • mimic actions such as talking on the phone • begin walking • use isolated words
1½–2½ years	Stage 5 Roles, Goals, & Language	Symbolic cognition allows for a new kind of intelligence. Children can • practice true language (by way of two-part sentences; rapid vocabulary expansion) • explore social roles (partners, leader–follower, giver–receiver, etc.) and understand simple goals (their own and others') • understand cooperation vs. defiance, "mine" vs. "yours" • use language to attain goals • use "no!" to define limits
2½–3½ years	Stage 6 Social Maneuvering	An advanced understanding of rules in social context emerges. Children can • test limits set by authority figures • use sentences that include connected ideas • understand simple stories • coordinate two-role relationships (allowing for rivalry, jealousy)
3½–5 years	Stage 7 Perspective-Taking	A massive shift in social cognition helps children see the world less subjectively. Children can • appreciate different perspectives and viewpoints • grasp the difference between appearance and reality • be aware of other people's thoughts or feelings (*theory of mind*) • exhibit accurate counting and alphabet knowledge • begin to engage in intentional deception

problems, like sucking continuously on an object or thumb, or keeping track of a moving mobile. More complicated problems, like reaching for an interesting toy in the right location and bringing it to the mouth, are simply beyond their ability until the next stage dawns at 4 to 5 months.

Stage 2
Actions & Outcomes: 4 to 8 months

When babies make the transition to Stage 2, their behavioral habits change dramatically. Because of a universal, maturational increase in their working memory capacity, from one to two units, they are now capable of coordinating (or linking) two simple cognitive entities: sometimes a perceptual image with an action command, sometimes two perceptual images, and sometimes two action commands. This coordination gives rise to a number of new skills. In the previous stage, it was impossible for them to track a moving object with their eyes and, at the same time, reach for it with their hands. They could do either in isolation, but they couldn't put the two together. Now, by dint of coordinating these two cognitive operations, they can aim their hand at a moving object and reach it! In a similar manner, younger babies were able to reach in the general direction of a stationary object, but they would often stop the action sequence if they were lucky enough to make contact with it. They were also able to grasp an object placed against their palms. But with only one unit of working memory available, they were not able to reach for an object and then smoothly close their hand around it when they made contact. Now, with two units of working memory available, one to conceptualize the reach, the other to conceptualize the grasp, reaching and grasping become coordinated. In the mind and in the world. Reaches are now conducted *for the purpose of* grasping.

These coordinations open up a brand-new way of acting on the world, and this change is so powerful, so dramatic, so transformative, that we can barely grasp it (no pun intended). By the age of 4 to 5 months, babies can reach out their hand *in order* to grasp the object, to have that object, that toy, in the palm of their hand, to feel its heft, its texture, and in all probability to launch a second intentional action: putting it into their mouths. Actions are now committed for the sake of their outcomes. In other words, babies can perform an action with their bodies that is intended to produce an effect; to alter what is being perceived by their eyes, ears, and skin; and to change the world as they experience it. Acting on the world for a purpose, that is, toward a goal, just wasn't a possibility up until now. That's why, in the Orienting stage, babies could be quite content to continue doing whatever they were doing: gazing at a mobile, sucking on a toy, or grasping a fold in their clothing. Now, babies are no longer content to just continue doing anything. What makes them happy is to launch a particular action in order to produce a particular outcome, one that is new, expectable, and desirable to boot.

Now, babies start to reach for everything, they turn their heads around rapidly to see what's going on outside their field of vision (by about 5 to 6 months), and they hungrily explore complicated scenes (like a room with several people doing different things), looking for something or someone in particular.

The shift into the new stage is dramatic because, with the capability of coordinating motor actions, and to imagine a perceptual change that is dependent on an action, they now become aware that the world is full of opportunities: full of things to do, to reach for, touch, grasp, suck on. It's as if they had lived in a cocoon and have suddenly hatched. The coordinations that babies master at 4 to 5 months are sensorimotor acts we take for granted. But the skills we use in reaching for a cup of coffee and bringing it to our mouths are exactly those that infants acquire at this age. We perform these acts unconsciously and automatically, of course, for the sake of achieving a goal, a result. But for 4-month-old infants, every bit of concentration is involved in the actions themselves, and nothing is taken for granted. The world is an exciting place! This is often the age at which mothers begin to complain about how distracted their babies are during nursing or bottle-feeding sessions. Whereas before this stage babies were content to focus completely on feeding, now they are constantly distracted by the pulsing, whirling, colorful world around them. They have learned that their actions get results, and they take great joy in manipulating anything and everything that is movable, touchable, and suckable. As we see in the next chapter, many of the goals infants pursue have to do with play routines. Babies now come to expect that their invitations to play will be responded to—by you! This can easily lead to disappointment when you're trying to say good night and leave the room, and that's why we advise waiting until the first 2 months of this stage have passed before you attempt sleep training. However, things change again fairly soon. By 6 to 7 months, the latter half of Stage 2, babies' reaches are no longer awkward and jerky but smooth and practiced. Now they get what they're after with relative ease, and this makes the world somewhat predictable, while conferring on the child a degree of self-confidence. This ushers in a phase of emotional stability and relative independence—a good time for teaching your baby to sleep.

Stage 3
Point & Click: 8 to 12 months

After babies master the basic skills of Stage 2, they enter a period of exploration and play that remains quite stable until about 8 months, and then things start to change again. With a further increase in working memory, babies enter Stage 3. Now all the interesting actions that they can perform become coordinated with a second set of actions, performed either by themselves or by another person. For example, prior to 8 or 9 months, babies do not know how to bring a distant toy within range so that they can play with it. Basically, they don't know how to use some intermediary action to facilitate the thing they have in mind. (By the way, even apes are ahead of babies in this regard. They are quite capable of using a stick to knock a piece of food out of a tree so they can eat it.) In a study that we performed some years ago, an attractive toy duck was placed on a cloth in front of the infant, and we waited to see whether the infant could pull on the cloth in order to bring the duck close enough to play with. Even with prompting and several demonstrations, infants younger than 8 to 9 months had no idea how to do it. They might get involved with the cloth and pull it, but then they would forget about the duck! By about 9 months, however, infants would generally pull the cloth, keep their eyes on the duck, and then grab it—a clear demonstration that they could link two coordinated action sequences. Another famous study was first conducted by Piaget with his own children. He placed a set of keys under a cup right in front of his infant son. Up until the age of 8 months, the boy showed no sign of picking up the cup to get the keys. Once the keys were hidden, it was as if they had disappeared. But by 9 months, almost universally, children are able to pick up the cup (often with one hand) and reach for the keys (often with the other). There is no doubt, when watching this happen, that the baby is removing the cup *in order* to get the keys—another example of Stage 3 thinking. Upon entering the new stage, babies look a lot smarter than they did merely a month ago. Instead of losing attention when something disappears from view, 8- to 9-month-olds go right toward whatever it is that's hiding it.

The shift into Stage 3 brings advances in the social world too, which are particularly important for sleep training. These advances are what gave us the name we've attached to this stage: Point & Click. We visit these changes in more detail in the next chapter. For now, it is important to show how they build on the same cognitive operations as the ability to retrieve hidden objects—the double coordination required to link two distinct action sequences. Prior to 8 months, babies will not follow the direction of a pointed finger. They will look at the finger, especially if you wiggle it around in front of their faces to show how exciting a finger can be. But they will not look at the object to which the finger is pointing. By the same token, they do not point. Sometimes, by accident, a reach will look like a point, but before 8 months babies have no expectation that you or anyone else will look in the direction they are pointing toward. So why bother pointing? All of that changes within a few weeks following the onset of Stage 3.

Now, due to an increase in working memory, the baby can keep track of two sets of actions: the pointing finger, which itself requires some attention, and the imagined action of another person looking toward the object to which the finger is pointing. Again, an expansion of working memory allows for more complex problems to be processed and solved. In this case, the complex problem is getting another person to attend to whatever you are attending to. This problem can be solved by pointing. But the most important change to come at 8 to 9 months is the infant's new understanding that his actions and your actions are related. This is what we mean by *clicking.* Babies now start to look at their parents for cues, and this is called *social referencing,* or they begin to vocalize *at* their parents in order to get their parents to *do* something: to approach, to pick them up, or to retrieve an object they have dropped from their high chair. All of these ways of connecting with parents require an understanding that the baby's actions and the parent's actions are contingent on each other. And this insight depends on the double coordination that comes with Stage 3. In the next chapter, we explain how these new cognitive capacities open the door to new emotional response patterns, most importantly, separation distress. It is these emotional responses that make the 8- to 12-month period a thorny time for sleep training, because saying good night inevitably involves the cues that foreshadow separation and loss.

Stage 4
Honing Skills: 12 to 18 months

Stage 3, like Stage 2, settles down and stabilizes within a few months. The next shift is the onset of a new stage at 12 to 13 months. The coordinations of Stage 4 do not increase greatly in complexity. Rather, they amount to new and more refined combinations of the mental events already coordinated, and the actions already available, in Stage 3. At around 12 months babies settle into a period of smooth, well-coordinated activities that keep them happy and busy most of the time. They put objects into boxes or other containers, dump them out, put them back again, and dump them out again. These "reversible" actions may be a way to *practice* the kind of coordinations that have been built from 8 months onward—practice them until they become smooth and seamless. And the automaticity that results from all this practice may be exactly what's needed to free up working memory further, paving the way for the next transition— a dramatic transition once again—into Stage 5. But one of the most important features of the 12- to 18-month period is the gradual acquisition of single words used to identify objects and actions—"Mommy" and "Daddy," "up" and "down"—words that refer to simple, well-understood aspects of their lives. Even the use of simple words requires effortful cognitive activity: namely, the heights of information-processing for a small baby. The child must pay attention to forming a very particular sound, synchronizing tongue, lips, and larynx, at the same time as she is referring to (and thinking about!) an object or action out there in the world. Simple utterances of this sort are really an elaboration of the social referencing—or clicking—that appeared in Stage 3. Only now, the sharing of attention is symbolized with a word. The advent of upright locomotion also takes place in the early part of Stage 4. There is no agreed-upon cognitive basis for this timetable, although theories abound. It may simply be that the muscles and balance system of the body are ready to take on a new and much more effective method for getting around. Because no dramatic cognitive changes mark the transition from Stage 3 to 4, this is also a time of increasing emotional stability and independence from caregivers. As we see in the next chapter, the growth of independence from 12 months onward marks the beginning of another optimal window for tackling a variety of challenges, including sleep training.

Stage 5
Roles, Goals, & Language: 1½ to 2½ years

The next general shift in cognitive development is one of the most dramatic transitions in the lifespan. In Case's theory, it is seen as the shift from one major period of development (the sensorimotor period) to the next (the interrelational period)— much of which follows from Piaget, who viewed this age as the dawning of the preoperational (or "symbolic") stage. In fact, developmental researchers of many different stripes point to 18 months as a time of unique and important changes in the nature of thought itself: instead of thinking about *things*, children become capable of thinking about how one thing *relates to*, *stands for*, or *symbolizes* another. The most fundamental example of this cognitive shift is the beginning of "real" language. By "real" we mean using not only isolated words to refer to isolated objects and features but also using combinations of words to refer to *events*. Language *is* the combination of words. And the reason language is the crowning achievement of human evolution is that it allows for a massive degree of cognitive organization and flexibility. By stringing together different words in different orders, we are able to represent any action, event, or scene, real or imagined. There is no end to the number and variety of situations in the world that can be symbolized by language, because there is no end to the possible combinations of words. Before 18 months of age, children may well be able to point toward the ceiling and say "up" when they want to be picked up. What they cannot do, however, is coordinate the word "up" with other words. So they cannot represent anything more complicated than a single, routine act. By 20 months or so, children are frequently able to say "Mommy up" or "Daddy up" to signify not only that they want to be picked up but also by whom. The additional communicative power that toddlers achieve by stringing words together is hard to emphasize sufficiently. Earlier, we suggested that the shift from Stage 2 to 3 was like building a bridge rather than trying to jump across a river. Now we might say that the shift into Stage 5 is like instructing someone else to build the bridge instead of trying to do it yourself. Language allows toddlers to name familiar things and events. But far more important, it allows them to express their wishes: that is, to name events that have not yet occurred but that they would like to occur. Language allows people to communicate, not only about the real world but also about the many possible worlds. With language, we can express our needs and desires and form bonds with other people who can help us to fulfill them.

The advent of two-word sentences at 18 to 20 months brings with it something called the *naming explosion.* Children's vocabulary now starts to increase rapidly, week by week. One week they have 10 words in their repertoire, the next they have 20, and a month later they have 50 or 60. This change is thought to reflect children's dawning awareness that words are powerful symbols—a highly valuable currency with which they can acquire all kinds of interesting things, not the least of which is a sense of connecting with and being understood by other people. But the linguistic advances of the second year of life are only one facet of a more general milestone in development. The beginning of symbolic or "interrelational" (connecting two relations) understanding, which is perhaps most obvious in language development, can be seen in other areas as well. For example, children begin to participate in games that coordinate social roles. A role (e.g., a helper, a giver, a receiver, even a parent or a child) does not specify any particular person or dyad. Rather, it is a symbolic entity that stands for a *type* of relationship. So, as with two-word structures in language, the coordination of two roles creates a role *relationship.* When a father asks his 2-year-old to help him sweep the floor, the child might come back with a broom and a dustpan, giving one to the father and using the other himself. *You do this and I'll do that, and the two of us will work together.* By the way, "together" is one of the words our boys picked up at 21 months, and that word speaks volumes about their understanding of social relationships.

Language really takes off around 18 months of age.

Other expressions of symbolic thought include children's understanding that other people have goals and wishes. Of course, a goal is not a tangible thing; it is an idea or symbol that can be inferred from behavior. Babies had some sense of other people as intentional beings (acting according to goals) prior to this stage. However, 18-month-olds begin to represent the coordination of two goals, or the success versus failure of a goal. They begin to try to change people's goals, help them to attain them, or, very often, challenge them and assert their own goals in their place. It is usually not until 18 to 20 months that toddlers regularly begin to use that most powerful of words, "No!" "No" means *I don't want to do what* you *want me to do—I want to do what* I *want to do.* It becomes important to say "no" when you realize that you live in a world where everyone has different, often competing goals. How else would you assert your own will? The word "mine" also appears soon after 18 months, as children begin to understand a primitive form of ownership. Once again, the idea of ownership refers to an invisible (symbolic) relationship between a person's sphere of control and some object that may or may not be within that sphere. To claim that something is "mine" allows the child to demonstrate some control over the world of valuable, desirable things.

> The word "no!" becomes a
> regular, and powerful, part of
> the new toddler's repertoire.

The stage beginning at 18 months encompasses enormous changes in the child's understanding of the world in general and the social world in particular, and it offers new tools for being an effective social being. However, as we explore in the next chapter, it is also a time of renewed emotional vulnerability after a period of confidence and relative independence. Because the child's bond with her parents is beginning to be understood in radically new ways, there is an increased need to confirm inter-personal closeness and thereby minimize insecurity. And there is a corresponding increase in the intensity of separation reactions. It should begin to be obvious that this is not a good age to begin sleep training, or any other change that promotes uncertainty about the parent's accessibility. At least not until the second half of the stage, when things settle down considerably.

Stage 6
Social Maneuvering: 2½ to 3½ years
The next two transitions have not been studied as carefully as those we've discussed so far, at least not by neo-Piagetians. However, findings from a broad range of studies point to several

fascinating changes in how toddlers think and act. The transition from Stage 5 to 6, at about 28 to 30 months (2½ years), spells major advances in the complexity of the sentences, stories, and rule relationships children can understand and manipulate. For example, children can knowingly either follow or violate rules well before 2 years. They know that throwing food is frowned upon, but they do it anyway, with a maddening glint in their eye, and they know in some vague way that cleaning up toys is a good thing. Two-year-olds can also be aware of people's goals and the feelings that arise when they are satisfied or obstructed. *Mommy is happy when I eat my carrots. My sister is sad when I hit her.* Yet they don't see rules and goal-seeking in relation to each other. Which means that they don't really get the *purpose* behind rules. By 2½ or 3, however, children come to understand that parents' goals and feelings have everything to do with rules. Rules are a recipe for making parents happy or angry. Breaking rules now involves more than just a display of selfhood: it marks a true rebellion, and that's an expression of real power. We believe this is one reason why the Terrible Twos often get worse, not better, at the age of 2½. But kids this age can also follow rules to make parents happy or to keep Grandma from scolding them. In sum, children can now follow rules or break them in order to influence other people's feelings. Hence Social Maneuvering. This level of social understanding, and its use for good, not evil, so to speak, may be an important start on the path of moral development—the acquisition of knowledge about what is right and wrong and the ability to choose accordingly.

The other social acquisition we emphasize for this period is a different animal, and one often seen as a monster: jealousy. Now is the time when true jealousy first rears its ugly head, because jealousy involves the comparison of two social relationships: you and me versus you and him, that other fellow over there who you seem to be quite taken with! The more attention you give to him, the less you have for me. That's the cognitive computation underlying real jealousy. This level of cognitive processing is exactly the same as that required to understand and manipulate others' feelings by obeying or disobeying the rules, and that is why it emerges at roughly the same age. We get into jealousy in more detail next chapter, because of its intimate connection with shame, feelings of inferiority, and other negative emotional states. In the chapter after that, we explore its implications for sleep training, and we find that bedtime issues have gotten a lot more complicated. It turns out that the success or failure of sleep training at this age will depend a lot on whether there is another sibling around to bring the green monster out of its closet.

Stage 7
Perspective-Taking: 3½ to 5 years
By the age of 3 or 4 years, the portrait of cognitive development gets pretty complicated, because different kinds of skills progress at different rates—and that's true within each child's repertoire as well as in the comparison between one child and the next. Social development will come ahead of other advances for some kids, and lag behind advances in language, or counting,

or motor coordination for others. Some kids can count to 100 by the age of 3 or 4, others have a hard time making it to 10 until the age of 4 or 5. But these differences in counting skills may have no correlation whatsoever with each child's capacity to share toys, or understand why it's important to take turns, or have his action figures ride on the backs of farm animals but not dinosaurs. This kind of *skill dispersion* makes development more complex, and so do the factors in the child's environment that combine with genetic factors to influence these developmental patterns. The rate of the child's advances in all the domains of development depends, more now than ever, on the circumstances of his world: the availability of toys, props, and learning resources; the match between his drives and interests and the objects used for play and learning; social factors such as family composition, experience with daycare, and parenting style; the child's language facility; and more than anything the kind of social and intellectual support provided by parents and other caregivers for learning in different domains.

Despite this diversity, however, there is one important change that occurs almost universally at the age of 3½ to 4 years: the acquisition of what is called "false-belief" understanding, which is an important turning point in the development of theory of mind. *Theory of mind* is a phrase commonly accepted by developmentalists to describe the child's growing understanding that other people have their own perspectives, their own beliefs, their own . . . minds. In other words, children acquire the theory that other people have minds—thus, theory of mind. This capability is part of a cluster of acquisitions, all occurring at about this age, that involve shifting perspectives, often from a more subjective to a more objective perspective, and that's why we call this stage Perspective-Taking. As emphasized by Piaget and his followers, perspective-taking allows the child to shift out of her own view of the world in order to look at things from another angle, the first dalliance with true objectivity. This occurs in a purely physical sense—inferring that dad can't see his wineglass because it's on the far side of the piano—and in a psychological sense—inferring that dad *believes* he finished his wine, even though it's plain to the child's eye that the glass still has wine in it. Once children understand false beliefs, they have crossed a key threshold into the social world.

At about 3½ years old, children begin to understand that other people have minds of their own and often think and feel differently than they do.

False-belief understanding is a cognitive acquisition that is evaluated by a standard test with many variations. The child may be shown two puppets, let's say Bert and Ernie. Ernie puts some chocolates in the cupboard, with Bert's consent, for later consumption. Then Bert leaves the room. At this point, Ernie says, "Hmm, I think I'll put the chocolates on top of the fridge," and the examiner places them in the new location. To make sure the child understands what's going on, the examiner provides a running narrative of these events, and ends by asking the child where the chocolates are now located. Then comes a pivotal question: "Look! Bert is coming back. Where will he look for the chocolates?" The child's answer determines whether he is deemed to have passed or failed the task. Typically, children under the age of 3½ say, "On top of the fridge!" After all, they know that the chocolates have been moved there . . . so that's the obvious place to find them. But sometime between 3½ and 4, children's answers change radically. After a slight pause, the child might say, "He'll look in the cupboard. He *thinks* that's where they are!" And he might follow up by saying, "*We* know it's on top of the fridge, but *Bert* doesn't know that." By giving this response, the child demonstrates an understanding that Bert has a false belief. The reality is that the chocolates are on top of the fridge, but in Bert's mind the chocolates are still in the cupboard. In other words, the child now understands that Bert has a mind that is independent of other people's minds, and in fact independent of reality. Bert has his own thoughts, based on his own perspective.

The ability to empathize begins at around age 3½.

This insight, so obvious to adults, marks a massive shift in children's social cognition. They now see each individual as an "I"—a distinct person with her own thoughts, subjectivity, even consciousness. And with this insight comes a whole string of linguistic and behavioral changes. Instead of saying, "There's a blue flower!" they will now ask, "Did you see that blue flower?" They no longer assume that everyone sees the same things, or that other people see things the way they do. The onset of false-belief understanding means that children are able to think in terms of what psychologists call *mental states.* They acquire *mental state terms* like "think," "know," "feel," "want," and so forth—which refer specifically to people's internal states, not to the states of the world. That's another first. Indeed, people have minds and each mind has its own contents, and certain words about how the child or parent feels are intended to get at those contents. Most important, mental state understanding opens the door to true empathy, the ability to see things and feel things the way another person might. It also opens the door to deception: children can lie with the knowledge that their parents' view of the world depends on their perceptions, which means that it can be manipulated. So they might hide the cookie bag under their bed, confident that nobody else knows it's there. Finally, it opens the door to some powerful emotions, such as a personal sense of shame. Once you know that other people have their own opinions, you soon realize that they may have opinions about you! And those opinions might not be very flattering. Perhaps they see something bad about you, but you don't know what that might be. You don't have access to it. More on these issues next chapter, but for now we can safely say that at this age, sleep training—which involves leaving a child alone in bed while parents go off to their own world—can trigger emotional uncertainties of considerable intensity.

At around 3½ to 4 years of age,
children begin to deliberately
lie to get what they want.

We have now completed our journey through the stages of cognitive development from birth to 5 years, emphasizing the most commonly observed changes in children's behaviors, skills, capacities, goals, interests, and particularly the changes in their interactions with other people. It is not a far-flung metaphor to liken these advances to improvements in computer software. Because, no matter how their brains are constructed, no matter how many cells and synapses they have at their disposal at any given age, it is the "program" run on this fleshy computer that determines what capabilities the child will exhibit. Luckily, for developmental psychologists and parents alike, upgrades in this cognitive software are scheduled quite predictably and universally. New versions come along at regular intervals, as a result of brain maturation, which itself is determined by built-in biological factors, interacting with the flow of daily experience.

For the rest of the book we use this timetable as a skeleton, and we put flesh on the bones of this skeleton by focusing on the sequence of expectable emotional issues and how they map onto cognitive development. This sequence of issues provides a second set of stages that emerge from the unfolding of mental capabilities at the core of cognitive development in combination with the input provided by other people—particularly you, the parents. That's why the timeline of emotional stages—the subject of the next chapter—will map onto the schedule of cognitive development directly. Then, we show you how these emotional stages provide a platform for understanding how kids are likely to feel, and how they cope with their feelings, when you put them to bed at night.

3

How Your Child Feels

Emotional Development in the First 4 Years

WHEN IT'S A MATTER OF GETTING YOUR CHILD TO SLEEP, it's important to know what he is thinking, but it's even more important to know what he is feeling. Many investigators believe that children's emotional repertoires depend on their level of cognitive development. An understanding of cognitive development helps explain why stages of emotional development appear when they do, by specifying the cognitive tools children have (or still lack) at each age for interpreting the world in a particular way— evoking particular emotions, and coping with those emotions when they arise. A detailed model of emotional stages that parallel cognitive stages was developed by Alan Sroufe, and we borrow liberally from his ideas. In Figure 2 (page 56), you'll see how the emotional stages correspond to the timing of cognitive stages.

Let's explore the impact of cognition on emotion by looking at the child's repertoire of emotional habits over two ages.

Imagine that you are 3 months of age (or, if you have a 3-month-old in your life, observe her closely). You don't have a lot of talent. You can't speak, you can't make organized gestures or any other movements, you can't obtain what you want by virtue of your manual dexterity, and you can't imagine how you might get other people to help you get what you need. You don't even know what you need. You can't figure out what kinds of things make you happy and what kinds of things make you miserable, at least not in advance. What you do know is that your emotional world flip-flops from moment to moment, and these oscillations seem to parallel the wash of bodily sensations and sensory perceptions that keep coming at you all day long. You experience moments of intense pleasure when you see your mother's face, especially when she is looking back at you and— joy of joys!—smiling at you. You know that she looks and smiles more when you make noises with your mouth. You're not sure how to make these noises come, but as long as they keep coming you expect that your mom will keep smiling at you, and you in turn will continue to feel terrific. You may also recall, though you can't think about it as long as good things are happening, that the world is often disturbing. When you feel pain, distress, or anxiety, they often tend to get worse before they get better (and you can't remember that they ever get better during the time that they are getting worse).

In a classic experiment designed to manipulate infants' emotions, Ed Tronick, at Harvard University, had mothers stop interacting with their infants in the middle of an interpersonal exchange. In this "still face procedure," mothers suddenly stopped responding to their infants' vocalizations. They stared, instead, at their babies' foreheads, without changing their expression, despite their infants' escalating distress. This may sound cruel, but the study was extremely valuable, because it simulated what happens when depressed mothers find themselves unable to respond emotionally to their babies' cues. The result was robust. Infants aged 2 to 4 months became very upset as soon as they noticed that their mothers had turned off and tuned out. These babies kept doing what they knew how to do: making sounds and movements in order to get their moms activated, with the expectation that the mothers' temporary lapses would soon be over. But her continuing inattention frustrated them further, inciting ongoing distress. This distress led, in turn, to a phase during which babies looked away from their mother, apparently ignoring her just as she was ignoring them. But eventually, if the experiment continued past a certain point, a state of apathy set in, suggesting the infant's own entry into a kind of depressive state.

This is not a perfect example of the impact of cognitive development on emotional dynamics: after all, children of almost any age would respond negatively to such an unnatural cessation of their parents' attention. But it does demonstrate that very primitive cognitive operations—the expectancy of a certain kind of parental response to one's own actions—can be the basis of an intense emotional reaction. All it takes is the violation of a simple expectancy, concerning mutual play or attunement, and the result is anxiety, despair, and possibly even depression. It also demonstrates that, even at the same basic level of cognitive capacities, infants can mount a coping response: in this case, to move their gaze away from their mom. There aren't very many things a young infant can do to reduce feelings of anxiety or sadness, but averting gaze is one of them. By looking away from their mother, especially at an age when anything outside of attention is soon forgotten, babies manage to stop missing her so intensely. They effectively disengage from what is painful, as a means for reducing their negative emotions. (This is a tool for emotional self-regulation that continues to work, often as a last resort, across the entire lifespan. Remember Professor Higgins in *My Fair Lady*? He simply ignored Eliza Doolittle in order to avoid the unpleasantness of falling in love with her!)

What might produce a similar distress reaction 2 years later? Imagine you are a 27-month-old infant. You can talk! You understand verbal discourse, and not only the meanings of the words but also, more important, the thrust of the communication. You understand that you can appeal to your mother for help simply by saying, "I'm mad!" or "I'm sad!" But over and above talking, you have a highly developed social understanding: you understand that there are "rules" that exist solely in the family. And you know that if you violate the rules, your mother will be disappointed or angry, but if you comply with them, you will make her happy. As before, your mother's happiness makes you happy (something you now carry around as an actual memory, easy to recall at any time). But you don't expect her to be happy all the time. So, at this stage in your life, your mother's silence is not a make-or-break event, as it was in Tronick's experiments. If you have just violated a rule, for example by taking a toy from your baby sister, then you probably feel pretty good as long as your mother is *not* paying attention. Her silence is a good thing right now. However, if you have just done something "nice," such as sharing with your baby sister, then you really want your mother to be paying attention. Now her silence hurts. The point is that the emotional implications of the situation are much more complicated than they were 2 years ago. And they are just plain different. Now, "the situation" includes context, and your emotional response is accordingly dependent on that context, which includes your own "good" or "bad" behavior in relation to your mother's attention—not just her behavior toward you.

Once you have begun to feel upset because of your mom's inattention, the cognitive abilities of a 27-month-old are available for alleviating the upset feeling, allowing far more control and flexibility than you had when you were an infant. Now, instead of looking away, you can put on a pout and *show* your mother how hurt you are. That's bound to elicit some soothing. Or, you can use your language skills for telling your mother what she missed, in order to get things back on track. You can even tell yourself, or anyone else who's listening, that the person to blame is your little sister, not your mother. It might be easier to toss the whole thing off if this is just another occasion of the baby messing things up. This sort of emotional *displacement* (Freud had it right this time—a bona fide defense mechanism makes its debut) requires some pretty sophisticated reasoning, acquired sometime around the age of 2½. And, like other cognitive skills, it is immediately put to use in *regulating* emotional reactions and making the world less painful. (Note that Professor Higgins, who could easily have been one of Freud's patients, also displayed this more sophisticated level of emotion regulation when he stopped ignoring Eliza and, instead, classified her behavior as typical of womankind: *"Women are irrational, that's all there is to that!"*)

This example demonstrates that the causes of distress, and the means for alleviating distress, are very different for a 3-month-old than for a 27-month-old. The cognitive software for understanding and manipulating the social world, and for manipulating the inner world of experience, changes radically between these ages. The same sort of comparison can be made between any two stages along the ladder of cognitive development. When the child moves from one stage to the next, and his mental software is upgraded accordingly, then the computations that trigger emotional reactions are different, resulting in different emotions, and the computations used to brighten or soften those emotions are different—and more powerful—as well. That is why it is so important to be alert to the changes in your children's cognitive and emotional development if you are to teach them new skills effectively and smoothly—skills that include falling asleep without distress.

> Each shift in cognitive development
> brings on a corresponding change
> in emotional development.

To review, each shift in cognitive development is paralleled by a shift in emotional development, because, at each stage, there is a new set of *reasons* for glee or distress, excitement or disappointment, and new *tools* for adjusting thoughts and actions to minimize negative emotions (and amplify positive ones, for that matter). In other words, each new stage of cognitive development brings with it a change in what the child understands, pays attention to, and finds interesting, attractive, and frustrating. It also brings with it new techniques for adjusting thoughts, emotions, and actions when the distress meter gets up into the red zone. Between them, these two sets of abilities retool the emotional world in sync with the milestones of cognitive development.

Now that we can see the links between cognitive change and emotional change in theory, let's explore what researchers have observed about the stages of emotional development. We will outline those stages, in chronological order, based on the work of leading contemporary researchers, and show how each of them depends on underlying cognitive abilities. That is to say, we'll explain *how* and *why* your child's emotional responses to your actions—routines, separations, reunions, and the like—change in predictable ways at each step of development. If you understand the reasons behind these responses, you'll have more insight on which to base your own methods for soothing, playing, and teaching important skills—including but not limited to sleep training.

> Your child's emotional responses to your actions change in predictable ways at each step of development.

Stage 1
Basic Regulation: 0 to 3 months

The period from 0 to 3 months is often considered the time when babies learn to regulate their basic bodily reactions, their

Figure 2. Cognitive and Emotional Stages

Approx. Age	Cognitive Stage	Emotional Stage
0–4 months	Stage 1: Orienting	Stage 1: Basic Regulation Stage 2: Interpersonal Attention
4–8 months	Stage 2: Actions & Outcomes	Stage 3: Interpersonal Expectancy Stage 4: Motor Initiative
8–12 months	Stage 3: Point & Click	Stage 5: Social Referencing
12–18 months	Stage 4: Honing Skills	Stage 6: Motor Practice
1½–2½ years	Stage 5: Roles, Goals, & Language	Stage 7: Social Negotiation Stage 8: Social Stabilization
2½–3½ years	Stage 6: Social Maneuvering	Stage 9: Social Comparison Stage 10: Family Membership
3½–5 years	Stage 7: Perspective-Taking	Stage 11: Self-consciousness

states—alert attention, quiet wakefulness, and sleep—and their physiology. These little beings have spent a long time in the womb, developing all the bodily mechanisms necessary to live on this planet, to eat, to breathe, to expend energy in motion, to coordinate muscles and senses so that motion accomplishes something, and to sleep when replenishment is needed. They have also developed the mechanisms for acquiring knowledge and skill—mechanisms that will allow them to pay attention to what is most important, especially the faces, voices, and actions of other humans. Yet these mechanisms are not put to the test until the baby leaves the uterine environment and arrives in the larger world—no doubt a rude awakening! Now each of these mechanisms starts to function. The lungs have to breathe, the mouth has to suck, the esophagus has to establish its waves of motion, the stomach has to digest whatever comes along. At the same time, energy has to be extracted from nourishment and used effectively to power the organs and muscles. Levels of arousal have to go up when it's time to be awake and down when it's time to be asleep. Hormones and enzymes have to flow to their targets according to whatever state of action is demanded. Eyes and ears have to become attuned to events in the world. Hands have to learn to clench. And, as if that weren't enough, all of these organic systems have to learn to function together, in synchrony with one another. Despite their vast complexity, bodies and brains have to start acting in a highly coordinated fashion. Systems have to be tuned to one another so that arousal, motivation, motor actions, sensory focusing, and the organs responsible for fueling them all become coordinated.

The first stage is dominated by the infant's need to regulate and coordinate basic bodily reactions and physiology.

This period of developing synchrony among brain, body, and mind is referred to as the period of "basic regulation" by Louis

Sander, a researcher who spent several decades observing infants and their mothers. Sander emphasizes not only the coordination of these systems with each other but also their coordination with the habits, states, and capabilities of the mother or other caregiver. Most caregivers in the vast majority of cultures are mothers. But primary caregivers can also be fathers, grandparents, elder sisters, nannies, and so forth. Our mention of "the mother" should be taken to include anyone who plays that crucial role. But why is coordination with the mother so critical? And if it is so critical, why didn't evolution build it in, as it did with birds? Why does it have to be acquired the hard way, through development?

Mothers in different cultures have very different habits of nursing their infants. According to Ronald Barr, mothers of the !Kung San hunter-gatherers living in the Kalahari (in Botswana) nurse their babies on average every 13½ minutes, for 1 to 2 minutes per feed, and this goes on for the first 2 to 3 years of the child's life. In West European and North American societies, periods of nursing are generally separated by several hours. But even within Western cultures there is considerable variety, depending on whether the mother is working or not, how many other children she has, and whether it is the mother who is even doing the feedings. Young infants have to adapt to these radical differences in feeding schedules. But at the same time, mothers, fathers, and other caregivers have to get used to each particular infant's needs and capabilities. Some young infants can last for hours between feedings. Others, because of digestive patterns or needs for soothing, are better off fed more frequently. Sander is very interested in how the infant and caregiver manage to adjust to each other's needs and capacities, since it's obvious that the field of possibilities is wide open—there is no "right" amount of time or frequency to nurse a baby. Barr has shown in many studies that the *quality* of this adjustment predicts the baby's biological and psychological health throughout his subsequent development. But your grandmother could probably have told you that too. We intuitively understand that infant–mother coordination is one of the most important predictors of a happy, healthy childhood.

> Coordination between mother and child in terms of feeding and soothing is crucial for healthy development.

Before 2½ to 3 months, it's difficult for parents to understand why their baby is crying some times and not others. As new parents during the first few months of our twin boys' lives, we were often struck by how much we felt we needed some rational explanation for what our babies were going through. To alleviate *our* anxieties. They're fed, changed, warm . . . then what's wrong? Why are they still crying? The simple and incredibly complex answer is this: the infant is working hard to become biologically regulated. His stomach reacted to something mother ate, he didn't burp at precisely the right moment, he got a speck of dust in his eye and didn't blink quickly enough, he's overtired, he's overaroused, he hates that particular rhythm of bouncing, and so on. But it's all happening under the skin, and so many of us new parents, through the blur of sleep deprivation, try to solve mysteries that can't be solved.

So how *do* we know when things are working out properly during this critical stage? The success of the Basic Regulation period is marked by the smoothness, predictability, and emotional ease with which the infant shifts from one state to another: from alertness, to drowsiness, to sleep, and back again. Each of these states is unique psychologically and physiologically, and each has its purpose. A well-adjusted infant–mother bond is demonstrated by the infant's ability to spend some time in each of these states and to shift easily to another state when the situation or bodily requirements demand it.

But there is another marker that things are going well in this stage—one that is gleaned entirely through the emotional tone of your interaction with your baby. A successful resolution of Basic Regulation is evidenced by increasing smiling, decreasing distress, and lots of direct face-to-face contact, as well as the baby's ability to turn off, turn away, and relax—or even fall asleep—between bouts of social interaction. At around the age of 2½ to 3 months, babies become a lot more attentive and social. It's as if they no longer have to worry about making their bodies and brains work properly and now they can have some fun being in the world. Also, due to their rapidly growing preoccupation with human faces, they become more fun to be with. The famous "social smile" begins to appear quite regularly by this age, and that is a true reward for parents' hard work over the previous weeks and months. It is also an age at which babies begin to go longer *between* feedings, especially at night. In fact, it is often not until 6 or 8 weeks that babies really distinguish between night and day. And by 2½ months they may sleep for 4, 5, or 6 hours at a stretch during the night, while still requiring feeding (and naps!) every 3 hours during the day. That means not only more rest for you but also more time to play, to coo and goo at each other, to gaze into each other's eyes with no other task at hand. Now there's an opportunity to get to *like* one another, instead of always working to satisfy needs.

> By the end of this stage, infants are smiling more, gazing longer at the parent, and relaxing more in their environment.

In sum, the Basic Regulation stage is a time when the child's body and brain systems become connected to each other, synchronized with the rhythms of parents and other family members, and coordinated with the conditions of the world she lives in, including the planetary rotation that produces day–night cycles. Because there is so much going on, so much learning, connecting, and synchronizing, and because the infant's progress through these challenges has its own natural rhythm, we do not recommend sleep training during this stage. Basic Regulation is a time to follow your baby's cues, not to impose a set of prefabricated constraints. Here's one way to put it: let the internal clock finish getting built before you try setting it. We review and elaborate these suggestions (and their rationale) in the next chapter. For now, suffice it to say that neither you nor your baby will be sleeping for long periods during this stage, unless you're one of the lucky few. Get used to the idea! That's the price we generally have to pay, the import duties charged for new human beings. But by inviting these delightful creatures to join us, and allowing them to adjust to our world at their own pace, we pave the way for a well-functioning human organism in a secure and stable relationship that will make sleeping easier in the future.

Needless to say, the satisfactory resolution of the Basic Regulation period spells great relief for parents. Not only is your baby more fun to be with in the day, but he is more predictable, more easily understood. The reasons for his physical and emotional states become more readily available, and that in itself allows you to relax and feel a bit more like you know what you're doing. And finally, now, after the first 3 months, your baby may actually let you sleep for a few hours at night! If you're lucky, sleep training may even turn out to be unnecessary, as some babies begin sleeping for 8-hour stretches on their own at around 3 months. Most do not. But even babies who don't sleep for long stretches may now have the capability to sleep longer periods than ever before. Because bodily systems are well synchronized and the infant–parent bond is vibrant and robust, the next period, what we call Interpersonal Attention, is a more resilient stage of emotional development. Sleep training should wait at least until then.

Stage 2
Interpersonal Attention: 2½ to 4 months

By 2½ to 3 months, and until about 4 to 4½ months, the baby's full-bore attention to people and their activities marks a new stage of emotional development. We refer to this short period as Interpersonal Attention, because it is a time when bodily habits, coordinated between mother and baby, have finally become consolidated, and the infant can now turn his attention to the most exciting things in the world outside his body: other people. At this age (which corresponds with the second half of the first stage of cognitive development, the Orienting stage; see Figure 2 on page 56 for a summary of overlapping stages), babies' limited set of skills includes grasping, sucking, and gazing at objects and people for long periods. But more importantly for our story, this age is marked by the initiation of *reciprocal exchange*, as noted by Sander, because it involves prolonged gazing at the mother and other family members, who inevitably gaze back at the infant. Babies now gaze at their mother, smile, coo, and delight in the ensuing changes in her face and voice. The mother, in turn, becomes fascinated by her baby's facial expressions, especially smiles, and especially the smiles that seem to be a response to her own expressions and actions. As described by Daniel Stern, this feeling of being noticed, being important, being a source of excitement and pleasure for the baby, is highly rewarding to the mother, who gazes at the baby while vocalizing in exactly the way babies find most interesting (called *Motherese*). The baby notices her mother's gaze and vocalizations, as well as the changing facial expressions that accompany them, and seems to know intuitively that they are directed *at* her. This interpersonal connection is practically irresistible to most babies, who will stare at their mother's face for long periods while cooing and gooing. From about 2½ to 4 months, episodes of mutual gazing stretch out longer and longer, and they become a fundamental source of excitement and joy for both partners. Scottish theorist Colwyn Trevarthen describes this as a state of *intersubjectivity* between the infant and caregiver. There is a sense not only of each partner responding to the other but also of both partners sharing a world in which "we are here together."

> The period between about
> 3 and 4 months is one of
> mother and baby "falling in love."

Many developmentalists see the 3- to 4-month period as the fruition of a "love affair" between the infant and the caregiver. But it is a love affair with all the qualities of a still life. It doesn't progress from moment to moment, and that's because babies aren't keeping track of what to expect, what happens next. This stage precedes the dawning of infants' ability to anticipate events, even immediate events, whether caused by their own actions or by some other agency. The cognitive software simply isn't there yet—not until the commencement of the Actions & Outcomes stage. That's why, regardless of how intensely your baby gazes at you, no matter how giddily she coos and giggles at the glorious sight of your smile, there is no disappointment when the interaction ends—as long as it is followed by some-thing else the baby can attend to. Even when left alone in a baby seat when you have exited the room to perform some errand, 2½- to 4-month-old infants generally will not fuss if they are dis-tracted by something interesting, at least not for a few minutes.

This may seem counterintuitive, and when one of us (Marc) was conducting his own research with young babies for his graduate work, he was more than a little surprised to see this lack of a reaction firsthand. The camera was on, the mother was instructed to "talk" with her 3-month-old as she normally would, and then, after 3 minutes of interaction, she was to get up and leave the room without looking back. A chime sounded at 3 min-utes, and the moms did what they were supposed to do: they got up and left the room. But when we examined the video record of the baby's face and body over the next few minutes, almost all 2½- to 4-month-olds showed the same response: they did noth-ing at all. They sat in their seats and found something to gaze at, a lamp or the leg of a table, or they clutched at the folds in their clothing, or stuck their fists in their mouths, or else tilted their heads back and made gurgling sounds, amused by the vari-ety of noises they were able to produce. The conclusion drawn from watching 50 babies demonstrate this pattern was hard to escape. Before 4 months or so, babies simply do not experience separation distress or distress at the cessation of an enjoyable interaction (though they may get distressed when alone due to other factors). And the reason for this is that they do not expect their actions to evoke a response from a social partner once the interaction has stopped. They do not *expect* a response from you, and they do not *remember* the interaction they just had with you. Their working memory is not sufficiently developed—not until the stage transition taking place at 4 to 5 months.

For these reasons, the emotional tone of the Interpersonal Attention stage is more robust and resilient than that of surrounding stages. After Basic Regulation, it will strike you as a period of diminishing distress, less inexplicable crying, and more contentment. A period of dawning interpersonal excitement, affection, and sharing, but without the sense of "what comes next" that is such a fundamental platform for all human interactions. Due to this resilience, this low-cost affection, sleep training is more likely to work now, from 2½ to 4 months, than before or after this period. But there may be some important drawbacks to sleep training during this stage as well. More on the pros and cons of this and other stages in the next chapter.

Stage 3
Interpersonal Expectancy: 4 to 5½ months

The budding reciprocity, positive emotionality, and sustained attention infants display at 3 to 4 months soon usher in a major stage transition in cognitive development and a parallel suite of emotional changes that are both challenging and rewarding. While reciprocal gazing may begin as early as 2 to 3 months, it continues to grow toward a climax that takes place between 4 and 5 months, kicking off a stage we call Interpersonal Expectancy. The climax of mother–infant reciprocity at about 4½ months is described as a key transition point by Margaret Mahler, an infant observer with a background in psychoanalysis. Now begins a

phase of *differentiation* of the infant from the mother, according
to Mahler, marked by a mushrooming sense of autonomy. It may
seem counterintuitive that a period of increasing mutuality and
closeness should lead to a spurt in autonomy. But it is no accident. The love, excitement, and learning that flow between infant
and caregiver during their face-to-face exchanges throughout
the stage of Interpersonal Attention push the infant into a major
developmental advance, a sort of blossoming of awareness that
results in a sense of a self—an *I*—who can act on the world *out
there*. Yet autonomy does not mean that the bond with the parent is over. Quite the contrary. Mahler emphasizes that the baby's
sense of a unique, separate self forms the basis of a new kind of
bond with the primary caregiver—a bond between two partners,
rather than a fusion in which mother and baby act as parts of a
single organism. Infants now begin to interact with their caregivers in a back-and-forth fashion (not quite turn-taking, as that
implies planning and waiting for a response). They may look at
their father's face, make a noise, a squawk or grunt or squeak
or any of the wonderful noises that come out of pre-verbal children, and then notice that their father smiles too and perhaps
reaches down to tickle the baby or manipulate his limbs in a play-
ful fashion. The baby may now squawk again, anticipating his
father's response, and so begins a chain of actions in which each
partner does something the other partner is likely to appreciate,
and each responds to the other in an ongoing exchange. Also at
this age, infants begin to initiate play and wait for the parent to
respond to them. So the onset of *differentiation* at 4½ months
is a time of both budding autonomy and increased interpersonal

engagement, leading to true play for the first time ever. The time babies spend gazing at their mother's face now begins to decline, but their attraction to game-playing skyrockets. Almost any kind of game will do, as long as it involves some repetitive, expectable activity. By 5 months, infants love the feeling of excited anticipation they get while waiting for the parent to swoop down, pat or tickle them, or throw them up in the air (a specialty of fathers everywhere, despite mothers' anxiety). And when they feel lonely, or bored, or tired, they still need their parent to be there, to pick them up, and to hold and nurture them.

> The infant begins to develop a basic
> sense of independence from Mom;
> they are no longer one organism.

This new stage of emotional development, marked by interpersonal play and growing autonomy, corresponds almost perfectly with the first half of Stage 2 in cognitive development—Actions & Outcomes (again, see Figure 2, page 56, for the summary of overlapping stages). In the last chapter, we reviewed the infant's new capacities to coordinate two events (such as gazing and reaching or reaching and grasping), due to an increase in working memory beginning at 4 months. And we showed how these capacities led to a new kind of approach to the world, one in which the infant's actions were propelled by a wish for and anticipation of some outcome, permitting intentional or goal-directed behavior. But what's the connection between the cognitive and the emotional changes at this point in development? The answer, we believe, is simple. Infants at 4 to 5 months act to produce an outcome, not only on *things* in their environment but also on *people.* Consequently, when they make a noise directed at a parent, they anticipate a response from that parent *as an outcome.* When they make a noise, and their mother or father responds, they connect the noise to the response. They coordinate these events in their working memory. And the next time they make a similar noise, they *expect* a similar response. Without the new cognitive software, this expectancy would not exist. Now, by keeping track of both parts of a social exchange—their own vocalization and the other person's smile, coo, or tickle—babies can engage in true reciprocity—reciprocity that goes beyond mutual gazing in a prolonged still life—and participate in a chain of actions, each of which is a response to a previous action by the other partner.

However, at the same time that these social skills are emerging, infants are learning how to act on the physical world in a way that is highly effective and highly rewarding. This was described in some detail in the last chapter. Instead of flailing their arms about and grabbing whatever their hands happen to touch, they can now direct their reach according to their gaze, and they can grasp an object just as their hand reaches it. With these skills, infants can reach for, grab, play with, and suck on the dozens or hundreds of things they see around them . . . and do so *intentionally.* The world of toys and objects now becomes highly appealing and compelling, drawing attention away from the reciprocal exchanges they engage in with their parents. So, the "love affair with the parent" soon has to compete with a "love affair with the world," giving rise to a tension or conflict between the interpersonal realm and the realm of inanimate objects. This conflict can result in unpredictable behavior. For example, one mother told us that her son suddenly began to avoid eye contact with her for 2-hour stretches at the age of 4½ months, a change that did not please her in the least. Not only was his attention drawn by the physical world, but his connection to the world of other people went through a phase of reorganization and his repertoire of responses was reshuffled accordingly. Yet the pull between physical and social attractions does eventually become resolved, for most infants, at approximately 5 to 6 months: the physical world generally wins out.

As we emphasize in the next chapter, these factors are what make the age of 4 to 5½ months a dicey period when it comes to sleep training. There is too much going on. There are strong emotional reactions to any opportunity for play. The baby at this age expects parents to be available when she is ready to play. In fact, just the parent's presence may seem to be an invitation to begin some new game. And when the parent is heard but not seen, the baby may call out, *expecting* a reply, and wonder why nothing is coming back. There is some evidence that separation reactions become more intense, at least briefly, around 4 to 5 months. As mentioned earlier, one of us (Marc) studied separation–reunion reactions around this age in considerable detail, and discovered that separation distress changes its meaning at right about 4½ months. Distress prior to this age did not seem to result from the cessation of a play episode or parental separation, as noted earlier. But distress *after* this age appeared to be contingent on the experience of loss or disappointment. This research was never properly replicated, and it is premature to draw any serious conclusions from this one study. However, for us, the study complements what theory and observation already suggest: that this is a period of rapid cognitive and emotional change, in which new cognitive coordinations permit the anticipation of interpersonal responses to the infant's bids. According to the principles we are laying out in this book, this would not be the best time to embark on interpersonal challenges centered on parents' whereabouts, such as the mysterious and often troubling separations that inevitably take place when they leave their baby to fall asleep.

Stage 4
Motor Initiative: 5½ to 7½ months

The infant's emotional life settles down quite noticeably in the next month or two, and indeed this stage, which we are calling Motor Initiative after Sander, is a period characterized by autonomy, independence, and resilience. From 5½ to 7½ months the new skills acquired in Actions & Outcomes become practiced and efficient (again, see Figure 2 on page 56 for the overlap between cognitive and emotional stages). And as they do, the physical world opens up to the infant in a way that we can barely imagine. The profusion of glittering surfaces, splotches of color, regular and novel movements must have seemed like a highly intricate decoration scheme—fun to look at but not very practical—to the younger infant. Now, the capacity to coordinate images and action commands allows infants to reach out, touch, hold, and bring to their mouths everything they lay their eyes on. This is why the physical world wins out over the social world. Infants have already learned pretty much what to expect from faces, fascinating though they are. But they have only begun to learn about what's out there in the physical world. Sander calls this the period of *infant initiative*, and we can think of no better descriptor. Infants now reach out into the physical world almost continuously, trying to grab what they see. They seem compelled, driven, to explore every object within their reach, first with their hands and then with their mouths. They touch corners, surfaces, indentations, and protrusions; explore textures with their fingers; and move their bodies in new and untested ways to get at things that are just out of reach. And then they suck or chew on whatever they can get to their mouths, exploring these objects with the tactile surfaces they enjoy most—their lips and tongues. The same period is described by Mahler as the phase of *practicing*. By this she means simply the repeated, energetic actions that infants engage in to get to know the physical world. Few infants can crawl by 6 months, but some can roll, creep, or move their bodies in the most remarkable ways to get closer to what they want to explore. The point is that everything they do is motivated by the excitement generated by objects in their environment.

Infants at this age are delighted to explore the world of things around them and are less interested in clinging to parents.

There is little to say about emotional development in the 5½- to 7½-month period, except that it is highly stable. The game-playing routines acquired by about 5 months continue to proliferate. These routines become more complex, more interesting, and more involved, but their fundamental nature does not change. Infants still see other people as playmates in simple back-and-forth rituals. They do not see them as agents who might be recruited to fulfill their needs, nor as other beings with their own habits and preferences. Perhaps most interesting in this period, infants' reactions to loss are muted. They may become frustrated if a toy falls on the floor and can't be retrieved. But their distress is usually short-lived or completely eclipsed by some distraction or other. And if a person suddenly disappears from view, they may gaze intently at the location where she was last seen. Or, they may gaze around the room, knowing that the person must be here somewhere. But at this age infants have no idea how to find what's missing. As a result, they don't try very hard, and soon their attention passes on to other, more accessible attractions. You may recall from the last chapter that it isn't until the Point & Click stage, beginning at 8 to 9 months, that babies actively seek disappearing objects. Until then, adults are constantly appearing and disappearing from the infant's view, whether we walk into the kitchen, go to the bathroom, or leave for work. The point is that if we don't show up again within a minute of vanishing, the infant forgets about us entirely and focuses instead on other activities or other people.

Infants around 6 months old are emotionally quite stable and resilient.

This is a very important point when it comes to sleep training. No matter how engaging and thoughtful your baby may appear, and no matter how good he is at noticing details he never noticed before, the 5½- to 7½-month-old infant does not search for people who have gone missing, for mothers who have just gone downstairs or fathers who have just gone out for groceries. And because they do not search, they are not frustrated by the failure that comes from searching for someone who can't be found. As we discuss in Chapter 4, this stable and relatively imperturbable 5½- to 7½-month-old infant is a good candidate for sleep training, because sleep training is all about vanishing parents. However, when babies near the age of 8 months, this window of opportunity disappears once again.

Stage 5
Social Referencing: 8 to 11 months

As we noted in Chapter 1, and as will be obvious by now, emotional development consists of a patchwork of stages, each with its own unique character, rather than a smooth progression of increasing or decreasing . . . anything! More than that, this patchwork has the character of a pendulum swing: periods of emotional sensitivity and social vulnerability are interspersed with periods of greater independence, tolerance, and stability. And the nesting of the first four emotional stages in the first two cognitive stages follows a simple logic: each cognitive stage is divided into a front half, housing a more sensitive period of emotional development (Emotional Stages 1 and 3), and a back half, in which emotional dynamics are more stable and resilient (Emotional Stages 2 and 4). Indeed, Emotional Stage 4, Motor Initiative, was a honeymoon in emotional development. The baby at this age was resilient enough to be left alone to play for long periods, happy to go on car rides, tolerant of sudden changes in routines, and, yes, amenable to sleep training. But now, at 8 months, as you might guess, the honeymoon is over. Now your baby is going to be more sensitive to your whereabouts, your comings and goings, your presence, and especially your absence, than ever before. Welcome to Social Referencing.

Like many other stages of emotional development, but more conspicuously than most, this stage depends for its character on a dramatic transition in cognitive development: the double coordination that begins with the stage we call Point & Click. Recall that this transition allows the infant to focus not only on one coordination (say, between reaching and grasping) but also on two coordinations (say, reaching/grasping with calling to a parent), permitting the parent to become involved in the infant's attempts to achieve her goals. Two coordinations (of perceptual images and action commands) are put together to form a single cognitive sequence, one that often involves embedding the baby's immediate goals within a communicative exchange with another person. What is critical about this cognitive advance for the emotional realm is that other people serve as an effective means for achieving what the baby wants to achieve, and this partnership produces a sense that both infant and parent are participating together in the same dance, sharing attention to the same object, or embarked on the same agenda. So, if the baby wants to play with an object she can't reach, she will look to the parent to retrieve it. She may tug on her mother's dress, she may point, she may look back and forth between the object and the parent. But one way or another, she will act on the parent in order to get the parent to act on the object—that's the double coordination that links the child's needs and wishes with the activities of other humans. That coordination is what allows the child to experience another person paying attention to her, to her needs, or to her goals. This "clicking" can be seen as the first blush of truly *social* knowledge and *social* behavior. And these moments of connection promote a powerful interest in other people: in their whereabouts, their goals, and the objects of their attention. At the same time, a dawning interest in other people ushers in the awareness of the many ways to involve them in the child's own pursuits. What seems to emerge is some sort of fusion between the baby's sense of how to get needs met and her engagement, interest, and attempts to influence other people's actions.

Let's add to this basic formula a number of specific skills and propensities that emerge around 8 to 9 months, also resulting from double coordinations in the social realm. We discussed most of these in the last chapter, but we review them again briefly here. Babies learn to point, an operation that combines a hand gesture directed at an object with attention to the target of the other person's gaze. They also learn to look where someone else is pointing, combining their attention to the pointing hand with their attention to objects at some distance out there in the world. Pointing doesn't make sense unless someone is looking where you're pointing, or you're looking where someone else is pointing, and it is not until this age that the infant's working memory can hold on to both parts of this equation.

> At around 9 months, babies learn
> to point, and they are delighted
> when their attention is seen to
> be shared by the parent.

Babies also learn to retrieve hidden objects. We discussed this in the last chapter, but in a nutshell the child can now keep track of the location of a vanished object, say behind some barrier, while at the same time reaching for the barrier in order to remove it. The capacity to retrieve hidden objects makes it sensible to search for them, just as the capacity to look where someone is pointing makes it sensible to point. The dawning of object retrieval was a cornerstone of Piaget's portrayal of this stage of development. And, as we will see, the 8- to 11-month-old's obsession with retrieving hidden objects is fundamental to a major change in social development: the onset of separation distress, based on an obsession with retrieving hidden parents.

Another social habit that emerges at this age is gazing at other people, usually parents, for cues as to the *meaning* of a situation. This is called *social referencing*, the phrase we've used to label this stage of emotional development. The classic experiment to test social referencing involves a piece of apparatus called the visual cliff. This is a Plexiglas (see-through) surface that covers an actual cliff—a drop of several feet in a plastic surface, often composed of brightly colored checks for easy visibility. The infant is invited to crawl across the flat, Plexiglas surface, which he very often does with little prompting anyway. Then he arrives at the cliff. Although there is no real danger, it appears to the infant that the floor is about to drop away from under him. Should he proceed or not? Prior to 8 to 9 months, babies (at least those who can creep or crawl) usually move blithely across the visual cliff, whether trusting in some divine protection or just plain dumb. But now, at the new stage, they generally stop and look around for their mother. Once they catch sight of her, they look at her facial expression. The experiment is usually designed with instructions for the mother either to smile encouragingly or to frown and look discouraging. Starting at 8 to 9 months, infants' actions depend very much on their mother's expression. If she is smiling, they proceed across the visual cliff. If she is frowning, they stop and treat the cliff as dangerous. The point of the experiment is to show that older infants decide whether to cross or not based on the parent's nonverbal communication. Their interpretation is contingent on the parent's social cues.

Beginning at this age, babies look to their mothers for information about the world before they act on it.

One of the most prominent infant researchers alive today is Joseph Campos, at the University of California, Berkeley. He theorizes that it is the capacity to crawl, rather than any general advance in cognitive development, that provides the baby with the insight to gaze toward his mother in order to get information about the physical world, its dangers and opportunities. And he may be right. The evidence so far is inconclusive, but Campos has devised many ingenious experiments to show how babies begin to learn about space, motion, and their own movement as soon as they are able to move independently—to locomote— usually by crawling. What we remember best about Joe's lessons on development is a videotape he showed us when we visited his lab several years ago. The video shows babies who, upon seeing their mother frowning, not only avoid the visual cliff but also hold on to the wall of the apparatus with their fingertips in order to pull themselves along the edge of the platform, appearing much more ingenious than we'd expected. That's how determined they are to explore the environment, Joe declared, and yet they still don't cross the cliff unless they get the go-ahead from Mom.

If we combine what we know about pointing and social refer- encing, both of which show up at about the age of 8 to 9 months, we get a broader perspective on what's unique about this stage of emotional development. Infants are entering a new kind of awareness of other people. Previously we called it "social." Let's go a little further, now, and describe precisely what we mean by "social." What babies now experience with other people is the advent of *joint attention*, which means an understanding that both the infant and the adult (e.g., the parent) are attending to the same thing. In the case of pointing, the infant understands that both are attending to the object being pointed at. In the case of social referencing, he understands that both are attending to whatever novel or uncertain aspect of the situation (e.g., the visual cliff) needs to be evaluated. According to Michael Tomasello, a world-renowned researcher into the origins of infant social cognition, it is this special capacity for joint attention that provides a springboard to another critical feature of development—the understanding of other people's goals or *in*tentions. If the infant can glean what the other person is attending to, she can also begin to infer what aims the other person has, what goals he is pursuing, what he wishes, what he wants. The understanding of others' goals is perhaps the bedrock feature of human social cognition. It is, more than anything else, what makes us *socially intelligent.* The understanding of others' intentions is the first step on the pathway to theory of mind, and it may be one of the fundamental capacities that autistic children lack. As we will see, this understanding of others' intentions is still at a preliminary stage at 8 to 12 months. It is just getting started. According to Tomasello and others, not until the period of 18 to 24 months do infants acquire a more objective and accurate understanding of others' goals, as part and parcel of the onset of symbolic cognition—the next major stage in Piaget's theory.

Putting all this together, what is the 8- to 11-month-old infant all about? Beginning at 8 months, we see an infant who is very attentive to adults in his environment, and in particular his primary caregiver. Very attentive! To the mother's actions, to see whether they can be harnessed to the infant's own goals. To his mother's attention. *Where is she looking? What does she see?* And to his father's emotional cues, as conveyed by his facial expressions. *What does he think of this situation? What does he want me to do about it?* In particular, we see an infant who begins to understand joint attention, who experiences himself as a social partner with his parent, sharing the same perceptions, the same world. And, perhaps most important, we see an infant who is attentive to his mother's and father's whereabouts. Now that hidden objects can be found, hidden mothers are impossible to ignore. They are to be searched for and found! If his mother has disappeared, where is she, and how can she be recovered? This is an infant who is aware that good-bye doesn't mean forever. This child not only is connected to his parents emotionally, attentionally, and intentionally but also sees them as never quite beyond reach.

This final point is crucial, because it is the fundamental basis of separation distress. As far as the 8- to 11-month-old child is concerned, a disappearing parent, like a disappearing toy, can be recovered. Usually by calling to her. Because that works. Intense, demanding vocalizations are common at this age, and their message is clear: *Where are you? Come back!* If it's a toy that's hidden, the two-part coordination required to retrieve it involves the removal of a barrier or container. But if it's a parent that's missing, the action required is to call out and demand her return. The parent who shares attention and emotional meaning will respond to that call, because her role is to be there for the infant, and her attention is synchronized with that of her child. The two-part coordination required to retrieve a missing mother is therefore the heartfelt demand, uttered, as often as not, in a high-pitched wail, to *get back here*! That's what removes the barrier. That's what retrieves the missing one. And sure enough, the few studies that have looked carefully at the timing of separation distress in infancy find a spike at about 9 months. Babies become more clingy, more demanding, and more emotionally aroused when there is any indication that the parent is about to leave, or when they look around and find that the parent is farther away than expected. Or when there is a stranger present—providing the springboard to yet another landmark in emotional development: the onset of stranger anxiety.

True separation distress kicks in at around 9 months.

This is where theory meets data, and we think it provides the most thorough and grounded perspective for approaching infant sleep issues. There is every reason for babies not to accept parental separation, to try to reverse it, fix it, through protests and demands. And that is what we observe. Not always, but far more frequently than in the previous stage, separation anxiety (fussiness, concern, low-key distress) and full-out separation distress emerge in this stage. The implications for sleep training should be obvious. This is not the time to try it! A new kind of relationship, based on a social partnership, is just emerging at this age. This relationship is built on a sense of connection and shared perceptions, and it is buffered by a growing distaste for separations and an obsession with preventing or alleviating them. Now is not the time to walk out of the room and say good night, unless there are already strong habits in place to ease this disruption. Any kind of novel separation, coupled with a display of incompatible perceptions, goals, and needs, will challenge the baby's new social sensibilities and very often bring on bouts of anxiety and distress. We elaborate on these trials and tribulations in the next chapter.

Stage 6
Motor Practice: 12 to 16 months

Just when we begin to think that our babies are entirely ruled by their needs, their vulnerabilities, their desire for nurturance, and their concerns for safety and interpersonal closeness, the developmental game plan pulls another reversal. The pendulum swings once more, and we are reminded that babies (in fact children in general) are just as taken with the joy of being free agents, exploring the world, as they are with their need for security. The period of 12 to 16 months, which we dub Motor Practice, is one such period. This stage has many of the same qualities as the stage of Motor Initiative, which transpired between 5½ and 7½ months. Both stages follow a period of rapid and dramatic cognitive change paralleled by emotional vulnerabilities centered around other people. Both stages are characterized by relative independence, autonomy, and emotional resilience. And both stages borrow much of their thrust from the pure excitement and joy of exercising a newly emerging motor capacity. In the case of Motor Initiative, the new capacity consisted of coordinations among gazing, reaching, grasping, and gross body movement, allowing the baby to explore and manipulate the vast array of objects in her immediate environment. Now, beginning at 12 months, the new game in town is upright locomotion.

Of course babies vary in the age at which they begin to walk. Some start walking as early as 10 months, others not until 15 months or even later. But 12 months is typical. And it's important to remember that walking is not the infant's first stab at locomotion. Crawling, which emerges for many babies around 8 to 9 months, also brought with it a new sense of mobility and freedom. But there is something unique about walking. You can cover more ground, a lot more quickly, while at the same time enjoying a bird's-eye view of the world. Margaret Mahler described the advent of walking as the period of "late practicing"—not a very evocative title. But Mahler was right in viewing the "practicing" infant as gleeful, independent, and fully enamored of the non-social world. This staggering, loping, adventurous little creature cares little about the respite offered by loving arms, until he becomes tired or hungry—or scared. Until then, he is a free agent, gliding about on a landscape of novel possibilities.

The 12- to 16-month-old is
curious and excited about her
new world of possibilities.

The cognitive-developmental changes ushering in the stage
of Motor Practice are not as dramatic as those that triggered
the previous stage. Babies are especially interested in reversible
operations, such as putting objects into a container and dumping
them back out again, or taking the phone off the hook and putting it back on again. But two advances are particularly relevant
for emotional development. The first one is the use of single-
word utterances to express simple ideas. These simple words
are mostly nouns: names of foods, "Mama," "Papa," and other
proper nouns, and simple prepositions and adjectives such as
"up" and "down" or "cold" versus "hot." The capacity to use even
single words to express one's wishes, goals, or thoughts helps
to consolidate the sense of a shared world that began in the
previous stage. Indeed, the capacity for joint attention, first seen
at about 9 months, might be the prerequisite for any language
use, because the use of words takes as its premise the idea that
both people are listening to the same sound and deriving from
it the same meaning. This is, after all, the basis of language. If
joint attention gives language its first boost, then language also
helps to extend and consolidate joint attention. In other words,
the shared meaning of simple words establishes for the infant
a sense that "self" and "other" really are paying attention to
the same thing. Baby shouts "Up!" and Dad picks her up. That

confirms, with utter certainty, that Dad knows what you want, knows what you are thinking about, knows what you intend. The second advance is one we have already introduced: upright locomotion itself. Though we don't usually consider walking a "cognitive" advance, a lot of concentration, practice, repetition, and refinement goes into the baby's efforts to get herself off the floor and gliding on two feet. This may require the same kind of practice that goes into many of the novel abilities of the 12- to 16-month period.

The main point is that the new capabilities to arrive on the scene soon after 12 months create a novel and exciting world for the infant—who can now properly be called a toddler. To be able to walk, even run, from place to place opens up great opportunities to explore the world. Now the child has taken her place as a bona fide member of the family, to whom the floor is no longer a prison, and for whom each room in the house presents a new invitation to play and explore. To be able to use single words to express ideas increases the child's sense that her wishes not only matter, are not only shared by others, are not only understood, but also have the power to harness the adult's attention and will. What the child says has tremendous impact on other humans, gets her needs met quickly and accurately, adding to her sense of being in command of a new set of capabilities and her sense of being socially important, central, not to be ignored. These acquisitions spell emotional confidence. The needy child of the 8- to 11-month period has vanished, only to be replaced by someone who is independent, confident, even proud, and who tackles the world with a certain amount of glee, optimism, and authority. As we spell out in Chapter 4, this happy and resilient child is solid enough to handle the challenges of sleep training. So, if you've waited this long, the 12- to 16-month period provides another window when sleep training may go smoothly and succeed with a minimum of distress.

Stage 7
Social Negotiation: 17 to 21 months

By 17 or 18 months begins the most profound developmental change to occur in the lifespan so far: a major transition in cognitive development, and a matching transformation in emotional development. This is the true watershed between infancy and early childhood—the hatching of the child from a preoccupation with physical reality to an appreciation of *relationships* between things or people. These include the beginning of language, relating sound patterns to events, the consolidation of a social relationship with parents based on an understanding of doing things together, and a sense of the self as a social being who is part of a family. This stage also represents a distinct swing of the pendulum back toward dependency needs and social vulnerability. Becoming a new kind of human being—a truly social being—brings with it enormous uncertainties about how to connect with parents in a way that threatens neither the child's independence nor his needs for safety and security.

In Chapter 2 we provided a detailed outline of three of the major cognitive advances of this period. Each of these advances relies on the coordination of two symbolic concepts, like the subject and predicate of a sentence (each of which stands for a person, object, or event in the world), or the success versus failure of a goal (standing for opposite outcomes of an intention or wish). Here we discuss each of these advances in terms of its implications for emotional development.

The first advance is language itself. Children shift from using words in isolation to embedding words in small sentences. The simplest of these sentences may be only two words in length, consisting of a subject (e.g., "Mama") and a predicate (e.g., "come"), or a verb (e.g., "Eat") and an object (e.g., "banana"). But the outcome is profound. By saying "Mama come" or "Eat banana" children are referring not only to a single object or isolated feature of the world but also to a situation, an event, which is a more or less accurate readout of what they are actually thinking, imagining, or wishing. The ability to string words together to communicate full, complete ideas and wishes, and the "naming explosion" that comes with it, provide the child of 17 to 21 months with the most powerful tool available for interacting with other people: true language.

What is so special about language? When discussing the stage of Social Referencing (8 to 11 months) we spoke of the dawning of joint attention and of the baby's sense of people as having goals or intentions. But these intuitions were still vague and ill-defined. The advent of language clinches the deal. When the child says "Papa come," and Papa listens and comes over to where the child is located, there is absolute assurance that both parent and child are focused on the same words and, more than that, on the *idea* that the words express. Their attention is synchronized and their intentions are synchronized. They are thinking about the same thing and they are sharing the same goal. This is a major improvement over the dawning of a sense of joint attention at 9 to 10 months. Instead of just looking to where the child is pointing, the parent is showing that his thoughts and goals are real, accessible, and incontrovertibly linked with the child's thoughts and goals. It's obvious that language provides an incredibly powerful way to achieve one's goals, and this is not lost on little people who don't always have enough skill or know-how to achieve their own goals. But in addition to getting her needs met quickly and effectively, the language-using child now begins to understand that she is a social being, a person, in a world of other persons, who share a matrix of thoughts, feelings, goals, and desires. The child finally sees herself as she really is: part of a group of beings who share a world of meanings and actions.

Now this realization in itself brings on both confidence and doubt. It's terrific to convey your goals to the adults in your life, to harness their attention for a moment or two. But it doesn't always work. Parents aren't always listening. And what if they don't listen? What if their attention drifts away again? It is typical to observe a toddler of this age saying the same thing over and over, or making the same demand repeatedly: "Mama? Mama? Mama? Mama?" . . . until his mother turns her head and finally asks, "Yes? What do you want?" Or "More, more, more!" with escalating anxiety, not knowing if the parent will actually fulfill the child's cherished goal of attaining more raisins for his snack. So even the glories of being a language user and the satisfaction of finding your place in the world of thoughts and actions shared with your parents have their dark side. Words have to be heard, and messages have to be received, or else the child is helpless, isolated, and worse off than before: a language user who can't communicate!

> The ability to use language brings
> on a new kind of certainty that
> thoughts and goals are shared,
> but with it come new insecurities.

The second advance of this period is the understanding of social roles, and in particular the coordination of two roles that are complementary. The child who can understand complementary roles sees himself either as part of the program or not. If Mom wants to dress you this morning (as she does most mornings) then your complementary role would entail pushing one hand and then another through your sleeves, and raising each foot to receive its sock and shoe. There is nothing sweeter than observing toddlers engaged in these complementary roles, and very often they are happy to play along. But not always. If roles can fit together, then they can also *not* fit together. This provides a hinge-point between autonomy and cooperation. The 18-month-old toddler becomes aware of this tension, because it spells a challenge for his sense of self. Playing a social role means submerging the self in a larger plan, for the larger good, but at the expense of doing whatever comes to mind. The result is a potential emotional standoff. Complementary roles serve to organize the fabric of a relationship in a way that pleases both participants. When roles don't correspond, somebody gets left out, somebody gets mad, or sad, or insecure. Which means that social roles become parts to play in the family drama, with distinct emotional consequences. Play your part, and everyone will be happy. Refuse and there's going to be trouble. Toddlers at this age can't formulate this logic quite so precisely, but they can sense the consequence of their refusal to comply. Hence a potential trade-off that pulls for autonomy at the expense of approval, or approval at the expense of autonomy. Not an easy choice for the toddler who loves both his independence and the feelings of closeness he gets from being "good."

The third cognitive advance has much in common with role relationships. It is the understanding toddlers gain at 18 to 20 months of competing goals. As we explained above, infants begin to see people as intentional agents at 8 to 9 months. And they manipulate those intentions with a pointed finger, or with a demand—a scream or shout—to get parents to do their bidding. However, this understanding of people's goals is implicit, intuitive, and lacking in clarity. At the end of the first year, infants have a sense that other people's actions have a direction that somehow spells volition, or intention, or desire, but that's as far as they get. To really understand goals as symbolic entities that can be influenced or manipulated, shared or blocked, one has to be able to hold in mind two goals, or two forms of a goal, or competing goals. That's what is made possible at this age by cognitive development. I can only understand your desire to pay for dinner if I see it in relation to my desire to pay, or your desire not to be on the receiving end. A goal is, after all, a choice between alternatives—a choice one holds in mind as a guide for action. At about 18 months, toddlers have the working memory capacity to consider two possible goals, perhaps competing goals, or to compare the success versus failure of a goal. So their understanding of goals is now explicit and objective.

At this age, understanding goals is as much a part of emotional development as understanding role relationships. Toddlers in this stage of development recognize that their goals are often in competition with yours. You want them to go to bed. They don't want to go to bed. You want them to eat their potatoes. They don't want to eat their potatoes. You want them to come inside. They want to stay outside. Congruent goals spell approval and positive emotion, much like congruent roles. But competing goals spell conflict, which can be the harbinger of anger, rejection, and the withdrawal of parental affection. (We know, we know: withdrawing affection because your child is "bad" is, well, *bad*. But parents are human. It's going to happen now and then, despite the best of intentions.) Given these ominous possibilities, why not comply? Why doesn't the child just shift his goals to line up with those of Mom and Dad? For two reasons. First, because he really does have his own goals, and he can't necessarily rewrite them. A toddler's desires are incredibly strong and not usually subject to modification. And second, because there is still this issue of autonomy. Perhaps it's a holdover from the previous stage, when the "practicing" toddler so enjoyed being his own agent. But in any case there is a real sense of rightness

to sticking to your guns and resisting your parents' attempts
to win you over. Perhaps giving in to the parents' goals means
that the child is inevitably relinquishing his. And toddlers in this
stage are hardly willing to do that! They like to be loved, they
like to please their parents, but they have no taste for ignoring
their own wishes in order to do so. And that's why the one word
we inevitably expect to emerge in the toddler's vocabulary at
this age is "No!" And why 18 months is often considered the
beginning of the Terrible Twos. We don't think that anyone really
understands the basis of this powerful sense of autonomy. But
nobody who has ever squared off against a 20-month-old doubts
how real it is.

Other changes in social cognition are part of this sweep of
novel thought patterns at 17 to 21 months, including a dawning sense of territoriality. There is little doubt that the declaration "Mine!" will first be heard during this period, along with
"No!"—signaling the child's understanding that possession is
nine-tenths of the law. It isn't enough to have a cracker when
you can hang on to the whole bag. That's another example of
getting ahead of the competition in the toddler's sense of the
world. All of these advances share the same flavor: they further
elaborate the child's understanding of a social order in which
she must participate, through the use of language and gestures,
in order to assume her position in the family and maintain some
chance of getting her way . . . at least some of the time. But
the emotional tone of these social advances should now be
clear: this is an age of negotiation! The child at this age is like

someone who has just joined a club that, once joined, can never be left. The club provides its members with a road map showing how the social world really works, bestows on its members the power to influence others in order to achieve one's wishes and needs, promises its members a profound sense of both inclusion and control. It is the only club in town—offering a social reality shared with other people who can communicate wishes, feelings, and desires effortlessly and quickly. It is a club that one would never willingly leave, because it offers its members a steady stream of not only resources but also true affection, understanding, acceptance, and love. Then shouldn't this be a time of social confidence? No! Because, though the toddler would never voluntarily leave the club, she never knows when one of the club managers will tell her she's on probation, she's breaking the rules, her status is being revoked until she gets her act together. So there is negotiation about how much you have to comply, to behave, to agree, to acquiesce, in order to maintain your good standing in the club. And that is a negotiation that the 17- to 21-month-old can't ignore.

The toddler at this age is somewhat of an addict. She wants nothing more than to continue to have access to your attention, your approval, and your support. As a new member of the club, she continually tries to make sure that her membership is in good standing, and that she can maintain the benefits that are her due. That's why this child calls repeatedly after her mother, even though her mother is only a few feet away. Or why the child is still whining for Mama *even when she's in her mother's arms.* That's why this child hangs around the threshold, unable to break away, when her father is talking on the telephone to a friend. That's why this child continues to test limits, to defy rules, to assert her own goals, and then make sure you're still there, listening to her, caring about her, and loving her. The child at this age, though feisty and independent, is also insecure. And her insecurity, while easily triggered by physical separations, as was the case at 9 months, is really about psychological separations: the loss of affection, understanding, shared intentions, and support. Children this age will cling to their parent, refusing to allow her to move out of range. But that's not because they are afraid they won't be able to find her again physically. It's because there is no better assurance of that parent's ongoing approval and care than the feeling of being cuddled up against her skin, or basking in her smile. We may never grow out of the need for that most fundamental reassurance, but it first makes the scene during this stage of Social Negotiation.

Although feisty and independent
at times, a toddler between 17 and 21
months is an addict for his parent's
attention and acceptance.

Given the powerful emotional vulnerabilities of this stage of development, and the importance of the social communication, complementarity, and understanding into which your child is inducted at this age, we see this as one of the worst times for sleep training. Now is not the time to reconstruct bedtime habits, centered as they are on proximity, shared routines, tokens of affection and support, and assurances of continued emotional connection. Now is a time to comfort and reassure, not to challenge or demand. We are not suggesting that parents have to comply with every wish their child expresses, at this or any other age. Many issues will require you to put your foot down, remove the child from the scene of a potential crime, or obstruct your child's acquisition of a precious goal, whether it's a fifth helping of strawberry jam or free access to Grandma's china. But bedtime is too special, too personal, for this kind of face-off. If you have already inculcated good sleep habits, you may still be in for a rough ride at 17 to 21 months. Good habits have a tendency to unravel when your child tries to implement some of the privileges of club membership. Stick with what works, and don't be afraid to demand adherence to rules that have already become routine and that have already proved their worth. But don't try to implement a whole new set of bedtime rules—not at this age. Instead, if you have not yet imposed a sleep regimen, you'd best hang tight and wait a few more months, until the insecurities of this age have begun to pass.

The 17- to 21-month stage of Social Negotiation is one of the worst times for sleep training.

Stage 8
Social Stabilization: 22 to 27 months

Just when the period of Social Negotiation is really getting to you—when you think you can't handle another bedtime, hear another "No!," or get through another 30-minute whining spell—things start to change again. They settle down. Club membership becomes the status quo. Your toddler starts to feel more assured that his compelling goals and needs will go on being met, at least most of the time, and that he will not have to relinquish them to remain in your good books. He starts to recognize that conflicting roles and goals will not be the end of him, or the end of you, and that your absences are temporary: you always come back. From about 22 to 27 or 28 months, that is, for the rest of the stage of Roles, Goals, & Language, no major new cognitive acquisitions come along to stir things up. Your toddler is able to take his new set of skills and build up a repertoire—of expressions, habits, gestures, ways of getting your attention, and ways to soothe himself when your attention is elsewhere. This period of Social Stabilization comes on like a holiday from the Terrible Twos (but it is a temporary holiday: they will soon return with a vengeance, we're sorry to say), and it may be a good time to begin or resume sleep training if your child isn't already sleeping through the night.

One of the main pastimes of this period is the continued growth of language facility. Like other cognitive skills, the acquisition of two-part sentences soon becomes so ingrained that it doesn't take a lot of working memory to "launch" this program each time. Rather, working memory can be put to other uses, like building up a vocabulary and putting nouns and verbs together in new combinations. Our son Ruben had to work hard to enunciate difficult words, like "helicopter" and "computer." When we would ask him to repeat "helicopter," it would be as much for the amusement provided by his facial contortions as for any serious learning goal. Ruben, at 22 months, would furrow his brow and jut out his lips, indicating fantastic concentration on the sounds and sequence of sounds going into this challenging word. Then out would come "he-co-li-per" or "puter-com-per." It was clear that Ruben was attracted to our lexical club, wanting to assert his standing by letting no word go unspoken. But getting those syllables in the right order was an effort, and Ruben could not put "helicopter" into a sentence with other words for several more months. This suggested to us that his working memory was stretched to its limits simply by holding the sequence of syllables in mind while working his lips and tongue to enunciate each one.

But why bother? Why go to all this trouble? Because talking is fun, and the more words you have at your disposal, the more seamlessly you can communicate, without thought, without planning, and let others know just what's passing through your mind right now. Meanwhile, at 22 months, our other son Julian would march around declaring "Wait! Wait!" with his finger held in the air in seeming admonition. He was practicing a fundamental coping response, and one that toddlers have a hard time with: impulse control. He wanted yogurt now, not later, and yet we wanted him to finish his carrots first. So we would say, "*Wait.* You can have yogurt *soon!*" "Wait . . . soon" provided a structure for containing his desire for another 5 minutes. But because this was a tall order, Julian saw fit to repeat the verbal structure, and the gesture that went with it, over and over, telling himself—not us, but himself—that there was a pot of gold at the end of this particular rainbow.

These examples show the 22- to 27-month-old toddler using the mental software of the Roles, Goals, & Language stage, which he has now been practicing for several months, to improve his facility to communicate and to alleviate his own negative emotions—in this case, anxiety—by taking advantage of freed-up working memory. The second of these skills is particularly important, because it demonstrates how each cognitive stage has a double impact on emotional development: downloading new cognitive software changes the way situations are interpreted in the first place, giving rise to new emotional constellations, as we saw in the last section. But it also changes children's facility for coping with those emotional constellations, as exemplified by Julian's raised finger and admonishment to himself. Really what Julian is doing here is using language and gesture to overwrite what he feels with an alternative construction: instead of focusing on the immediate desire for yogurt, he is focusing on a division drawn in time, delineating a "before" and an "after." The *before* is a time to wait; the *after* is a time to get the goods you've been longing for. The way these two-part episodes fit together, and the declaration of "Wait" that stands for their connection, epitomizes how toddlers use the symbolic coordinations of the Roles, Goals, & Language stage to reconfigure reality, making their needs less oppressive and compelling.

Beyond this practice of symbolic constructions—both those shared with others and those directed at the self—there are no major new acquisitions during this period. This is a time of consolidation, increasing social facility, increasing social confidence, and a partial return to the freewheeling, easy sense of self that characterized the stage of Motor Practicing. Toddlers' anxiety about separations diminishes during this time, and some of their stubbornness—not all, but some—gets folded back into the pleasure they get from cooperating with others. As we point out again in Chapter 4, individual differences start to play a larger role in parents' decisions and successes with sleep training when children pass the age of 2 years. However, all other things being equal, this 6-month period should offer you one more chance to get sleep training ironed out, so that all of you can appreciate the many joys of toddlerhood without the exhaustion that some-times plagues the families of young children.

Stage 9
Social Comparison: 28 to 36 months

The next stage of emotional development, from roughly 28 months (about 2½ years) to roughly 36 months (3 years), gets its name from two new constellations: the ability to interact with oth-ers based on a prediction of how one's behavior affects them, and the first glimmerings of jealousy. Let's discuss the first of these. According to Judy Dunn, a prolific researcher into the social side of early childhood, children this age begin to coordinate their newfound knowledge of people's goals with their growing aware-ness of household rules. We show throughout this book that new cognitive capacities are paralleled by advances in emotional development, and indeed that's the case here. At the age of about 28 months, on average, the next cognitive stage, Social Maneuvering, begins to upgrade children's mental capacities. Toddlers become capable of a double coordination of the symbolic units now held in mind. Taking one coordinated social concept, the notion of a rule that can be obeyed or violated, and linking it with a second one, the concept that happiness depends on achieving one's goals, allows the child significantly more insight and control. Because parents' goals demand that she follow the rules, the child can now understand how accepting or breaking rules asserts her own power over your goals, and hence your emotional states—no small advance in the diplomatic halls of family life. In fact, this understanding provides the child with a new level of social sophistication, social influence, and capacity for manipulation. Heaven help you! The Terrible Twos (Part Two) have now descended.

Toddlers will now test the limits, not only to see what they can get away with, not only to satisfy their basic need to assert independence but also to go a step further: to see how much social influence they really have. They will find a way to touch and eventually ruin or ingest whatever you least want them to handle: the kitchen knives, the computer, the bottles of detergent beneath the sink. With great concentration they will find a way to engage in the forbidden behavior as soon as you enter the room. But why waste this potentially hazardous action on a parent who isn't paying attention? Why do they do it? What could possibly motivate this Machiavellian twist? This isn't because they are truly evil—although we sometimes wonder. This isn't because they really want to wreck your day or be rushed to the hospital. It's because they need to know how much control they have over the thing that matters most: how other people are feeling. And they need to understand what lies behind bad emotions as well as good ones. What they are exploring is the background logic of the emotional lives of those they love and depend on. If you suddenly had access to that kind of information, for the first time in your life, wouldn't you dive in?

But the toddler's newfound capacity to be so influential—and such a pest!—is offset by another coordination that can be deeply painful. During the stages of Social Negotiation and Social Stabilization, toddlers were capable of understanding that their hopes of getting their wishes met depended on their ability to capture and hold their parent's attention. They left no stone unturned in their efforts to get you to pay attention to them, by repeated calls, interruptions, or demands. At that age they were also capable of seeing how parents would often pay attention to other things and other people, following their own mysterious whims. They didn't have to pay attention to you if they didn't want to! Toddlers of this age could see that their mom was helping their dad, or their dad was helping their mom, and they may have had a vague sense that they were out of the picture for the duration of that episode. But with Cognitive Stage 6, which permits a double coordination, the toddler's bids for attention, and his ability to capture it by force, can now be *coordinated* with his understanding that you are attending to someone else and helping *him* achieve *his* needs. This is the cognitive basis for jealousy. If I see that my need for your help or attention is in competition with that of someone else, say, my little sister or brother, and if I see that you are helping them instead of helping me, then I can infer that their hold on you, their capacity to attract you, directly takes away from mine. Your wish or your decision to bestow your attention on the other person takes it away from me. That makes my sister my rival! Anything you do for her might be at the expense of what you do for me. And this includes not only rewarding her with some sort of immediate help, a soothing word or a boost into her chair, but also the larger thrust of your preferences, who you really like, or love, the most. *Why are you helping her and not me? Do you like her more? Is she cuter than me?*

> Children experience their
> first painful pangs of real
> jealousy at around 2½ years old.

Jealousy is certainly one of the most painful of emotions. Once it is let loose in the child's mind, it seems to have the capacity to infect her thoughts and feelings, like a virus that self-replicates and makes the person sick. Nobody knows why it is so powerful, but we have all felt its sting. Nancy Friday, a brilliant writer who combines psychoanalytic and feminist principles in her work, shows how jealousy is inextricably coupled with feelings of shame and self-doubt. If the child feels that somebody else is more worthy of a parent's attention, care, even love, then she cannot help but see herself as somehow inferior. *Why her and not me? Am I ugly? Am I bad? Don't you love me anymore?* Not all children feel jealousy, and corresponding emotions of shame and self-doubt, with the same intensity. Not at all. The factors that determine how sharply this knife cuts into the psyche must include individual differences in personality and temperament, on one hand, and family constellation on the other. Some children are just more sensitive to the loss of affection, or even the outright rejection, that all children feel from time to time. Those children will certainly be more prone to jealousy. But you will probably already have seen your child's true colors with respect to "separation sensitivity," as it's called by David Kramer, during the stage of Social Negotiation, especially if bedtime rituals weren't going so smoothly at that age. Nevertheless, even the most sensitive child is less likely to feel jealousy if there is no sibling with whom to compete.

The 2½-year-old is particularly prone to jealousy if a new baby has shown up in the last 3 to 12 months. After all, there was no competition until now. And the little baby is so . . . cute. And you spend an awful lot of time with her, you carry her around everywhere, you seem entranced by her, over the top with all your cooing and gooing. What's that all about? The 2½-year-old now has the cognitive capacity to register competition and the emotional inclination to feel jealous when left out of the action. And now there's this little bundle of . . . protoplasm . . . that seems to take precedence over his needs 90 percent of the time. This is the best recipe for jealousy in many families. We don't know of a cure for jealousy, but as parenting books and common sense will advise you, the best approach may be to make time for your older child, to reassure him about his specialness, to show him, as well as tell him, how much you love him, and to explain to him that babies need a lot of help because they are so helpless. You can also enlist your toddler's help with the baby, while commenting on his prowess. This will ease the sting. And then you can try to enlist a regular babysitter for the next 6 months to get you through the roughest patch.

> The 2½-year-old is particularly prone to outbursts of jealousy if a new baby has just come on the scene.

To recapitulate, the stage of Social Comparison brings with it two new emotional specialties. First is the child's ability to manipulate your feelings by challenging your goals, violating household rules, and otherwise defying you at every turn, in order to learn about her social power and its impact on the emotional world of the family. Second is the child's proclivity to jealousy, and its tendency to fester and grow into a solid conviction that she is to be left out and slighted because she is generally unimportant or even inferior. There are enormous differences in both these outcomes from child to child. Jealousy is particularly variable, differing as it does in frequency and intensity according to both personality and family constellation factors. Because of this variability, our advice about sleep training must be buffered by your assessment of your own child's vulnerabilities and capacities at this and future ages. But if we had to lay bets, we'd say this is not an optimal age for sleep training, for two reasons. First, because your child's preoccupation with her social influence in relation to your moods and emotions may exacerbate her reactions to a change in bedtime habits. A new sleep regimen is something she can't control, and that may challenge her fundamental need to influence your emotions. Second, and perhaps more important, it's because your child's capacity for jealousy can paint any unexplained separation in the bleakest of hues. Separations are, once more, too powerful to introduce during periods of emotional vulnerability and doubt. More on this in the next chapter. But for now, our advice is to think carefully about the kind of kid you are dealing with. And if she is vulnerable to jealousy, shame, and self-doubt, don't rock the boat at bedtime. Wait a few more months.

Stage 10
Family Membership: 3 to 3½ years

As development continues to unfold in the third year of life, it becomes harder and harder to paint a unitary picture of emotional issues and concerns that applies to most children. The "average" child simply disappears over time, if it ever really existed. By this we mean that younger children's development follows a path of expectable stages at expectable ages that pretty accurately portrays most kids. They follow the sequence of cognitive and emotional changes with sometimes uncanny precision, as far as timing is concerned, and their abilities and habits fit nicely with the average picture for that age. But the older children get, the more they deviate from the norm in one way or another. The timing of changes begins to vary more and more, and so does the substance of these changes. Some children will follow one path of development, showing, say, a lot of defiance, jealousy, and negativity. Others will be more mellow, more content, and more concerned with cooperation than self-assertiveness.

> The older the child, the more
> likely it is that he won't fit a
> universal stage description.

The fact that children become more and more distinct from one another makes sense. The reason, according to Robert B. McCall, a scholar who advanced theories about infant development during the 1970s and 1980s, is that development has to be as "normal" as possible early on, so that children (and other animals) can accomplish what they need in order to survive. Too much deviation from the norm spells disaster. Most of the infant's behaviors are necessary to achieve the basic functions of physiological coordination, motor coordination, social engagement, protection, and nurturance. But once these basic functions are established, there's more room for variety, for individuality, for exploring the options. There are only a few ways to suck, to reach and grasp, to manipulate physical objects, only a few viable schedules for feeding and sleeping, only a few ways to give and receive affection in the first year. By the second and third year, however, there are many ways to interact with the physical and social worlds. Individual styles, temperament characteristics, and unique responses to different family environments take up more and more of the spotlight. There are dozens of ways to speak, to eat, to express one's discontent or one's happiness, and all of them end up *working*, one way or another. These variations take root in the world of the family. Parents adapt. And individual styles crystallize into stable human personalities. So, the older the child, the more we have to look at his individual profile instead of an age-based average in order to come up with an accurate description.

The period of Family Membership, from about 3 to 3½ years, occupies the second half of Cognitive Stage 6, Social Maneuvering. Not a lot of new cognitive capacities appear, there are no major changes in the toddler's basic thinking or orientation to the social world, but there are many minor changes, as certain abilities and habits get practiced and strengthened and others disappear. These variations are really the hallmark of this age. There is so much variation, in fact, that we cannot give you much of a picture of what to expect. We discuss individual differences in some detail at the end of this chapter. Let's focus now on what many, if not most, kids do have in common at this age.

First, they calm down. We call this the stage of Family Membership because children now accept their status as fully functioning members of the family. They know the rules, they have the capability to follow them, and they are not driven to test the limits in the ways younger children were. They're smarter about emotions—both their own and other people's. They know what kinds of events cause anger and distress, and they can adjust their behavior, and sometimes the behavior of others, to minimize these negative emotions. They can "be nice" on purpose to make you happy, or they can play on your sympathies when they need your approval. And they can follow the rules in order to maintain their status as family members in good standing. They are better at coping with or *regulating* their emotions. For example, impulse control was the biggest single challenge to the 2-year-old. But by the age of 3, children are able to wait until they blow out the candles before opening their presents. They are able to stop themselves from grabbing someone else's toy, to avoid getting in trouble. They're able to bite back on their anger before they hit or kick. And of course that makes them much better playmates. Children of this age start to play together in earnest. And although their play still is not truly cooperative, it's surprising how easily they can weave their own play themes together with those of other kids.

> By 3 to 3½ years, the child becomes adept at coping with his intense emotions and dampening them when necessary.

Children at this age have enormous verbal facility compared to children even 6 months younger. They use more words, in more complex sentences, but nearly all their speech is about social activities, events, and stories, using well-practiced "scripts" that are familiar and evocative. Three-year-olds also love to hear stories, and bedtime is an excellent time to devote to the child's favorite books. Those verbal talents come in handy when children have to share, or to wait their turn, or play with someone else, or just talk to their stuffed animal because they need some-one to talk to and everyone else is busy. The same verbal abili-ties also usher in a major acceleration in socio-dramatic play. Pretend games, where dinosaurs face off against each other, do battle, or wash the dishes together, or even have babies together, now flourish. Children of this age don't need as much adult con-tact because they are often quite happy to play with their ani-mals and dolls, where they can enact whatever scenarios interest them without having to get someone else involved. Each animal and doll has its own voice, its own position in the social hierar-chy, and even its own personality. And the personalities they bestow on their animals and dolls, the love they feel for them, provide an additional means for coping with emotions such as loneliness and separation anxiety. It is very common for 3-year-olds to have one or more favorite animals or dolls to go to bed with. The company of those beloved creatures, and the endless conversations they share with them, provide more resilience for coping with all household routines, including bedtime.

The 3-year-old is a relatively social, resilient child.

In sum, the Family Membership stage is often a happy time in the life of young children. Before the coming of false-belief understanding, which we discuss in the next section, they are not terribly prone to shame. While there is considerable varia-tion from child to child at this age, most 3-year-olds don't worry about what others think of them, and they often assume their parents' approval without much in the way of proof. They are not, as a rule, insecure. They are chatty and social. They love to interact through drawn-out conversations with real and imagined others, and they rarely feel lonely or left out. For these reasons, the 3- to 3½-year-old child is relatively malleable and resilient when it comes to accepting new rules and other emotional challenges. This is therefore a reasonable age to begin sleep training, if you have not already done so. In fact, it may well be the last age at which sleep training can be introduced without being accompanied by a host of mixed emotions and worries. And furthermore, the 3-year-old's attachment to stuffed animals will help her through periods of loneliness at bedtime and throughout the night. Of course it's very likely that by now you've already introduced some kind of bedtime ritual or regimen. But if it isn't working the way you'd like it to, if Jenny is still waking you up for a glass of water three times a night, then the age of 3 years is a good time to make the needed adjustments.

Stage 11
Self-Consciousness: 3½ to 4 years

The last pendulum swing we cover in this book takes place for most children at 3½ to 4 years of age. As described in the last section, individual variability is now the rule. Children's styles, temperaments, and personalities promote a wide spectrum of differences in language and social development, in habits of self-control, and in interpersonal skills ranging from toilet training to cooperative play. Children are now feeling like members in good standing in their families. They are so attuned to the social rituals of family life that they lead their toy animals and dolls through the same routines, cajoling them to be good, to share their toys, to listen to their parents—in short, to conform to the same rules that preoccupy *them*. But they now have the capabilities to be cooperative and obedient. They have developed the critical skills of impulse control, and they can use these skills to ward off or modify their feelings of anger, frustration, greed, and jealousy. Things are going well for the average child at this age. And then along comes another cognitive advance, rocking the boat once more.

When we described the cognitive changes of this age in the last chapter, we noted that developmentalists now tend to focus on particular domains of development: cross-domain or general changes in development (the kind we saw at 18 to 20 months) just aren't clearly evident by this age. However, one of the most important changes, usually observed at 3½ to 4 years, is broad enough to apply to some rather diverse features of children's social cognition: that is, perspective taking. We described this as the capacity to shift one's perspective (or to see that another person can shift her perspective) in order to see things from a different point of view—sometimes a more objective point of view. And one particularly important aspect of perspective taking takes place underneath the skin, in the psychological realm of thoughts, beliefs, and consciousness itself: false-belief understanding—the last major milestone in the acquisition of theory of mind. As you may recall, theory of mind is the understanding that other people have their own goals, feelings, internal states, thoughts, and opinions. In short, they have minds of their own, and the contents of those minds are very often different from the contents of one's own mind. False-belief understanding marks the culmination of theory of mind: the child can now predict that other people will believe whatever they perceive through their own senses, regardless of whether it's true or false. Many studies have demonstrated that 4-year-old children understand this basic principle of human perception, while 3-year-olds do not. By the age of 3½ to 4, children can predict that a puppet will look for hidden chocolates where the puppet thinks they are located—where he last saw them hidden—rather than in a new location where they were hidden a second time, outside this puppet's awareness. When children can separate their own beliefs from the beliefs of others, they have undertaken a remarkable shift in social understanding. They have now begun to glean that each mind is like a chamber filled with its own perceptions of the world, and no two minds need ever see the world in the same way.

Understanding that your parents have minds of their own can be quite a shock to the 3- to 4-year-old child. Up until now, you took it for granted that your mom saw things the way you did. In fact, you didn't have to explain to her how you saw things, because there was only one way to see things: the way they really are. Now that people's beliefs are seen to be private affairs, carried around in their own heads and not accessible to others, a number of issues have to be worked out. One of us (Marc) tells the story of his daughter Zoe, who rode on the back of his bicycle to nursery school every day from her third birthday on. She would typically point to interesting sights as they rode by, saying, "That flower is blue! That boy has a funny hat!" and so forth. Around the age of 3 years and 4 months, however, her language changed. She began to phrase these comments as questions rather than statements: "Did you see the blue flower? Do you think that hat is funny?" She was clearly conceding that his reality was not the same as hers. But other changes were less cheerful in tone. At exactly the same age, Zoe would be sitting at the table eating her cereal when her father came downstairs, and Zoe would shout, "Don't look at me!" while turning her head away or hiding behind her cereal box. What could have prompted such outbursts? If your parents have minds of their own, and if you don't know what's inside them, then you might well worry. They might be looking at you, and they might be thinking . . . anything! They might be thinking that you just spilled your cereal, or that you were supposed to wait, or more generally, that you're a bad, selfish little girl. How would you know?

In this way, false-belief understanding can be a ticket to a new suite of insecurities. A private mind, with its own thoughts and beliefs, might harbor thoughts about you that aren't very nice. This conjecture has been reinforced for us by many anecdotes. Parents of 3½-year-old children would tell us that their daughter suddenly stopped letting them hear her sing. "Go away! Don't listen!" Or "Don't look at me!" Or "Go away until I tell you!" This is often also the age when children suddenly stop letting their parents help them at the potty, if they've been potty-trained for a while. These reactions suggest extreme self-consciousness. These kids apparently worried about being seen, or being heard, because there was something about themselves that might not live up to such scrutiny. Something unpleasant, or greedy, or bad. In fact, false-belief understanding seemed to bring about a spurt of intense shame reactions.

To test this assumption, one of the authors of this book, Marc, conducted a study several years ago with Carla Baetz, his graduate student at the time. To see whether false-belief understanding brought about shame reactions, Carla went to the houses of 3- to 4-year-old children and conducted a shame-induction task. The task itself was on the sneaky side, but psychologists often trick their subjects in the name of science. Carla pulled on the legs of an elasticized doll and encouraged the child to do the same to its arms. What the poor child didn't know was that the doll had been tampered with: one of its arms had been cut so it was ready to come off, and a little too much tension was sure to break it. Indeed, the enthusiastic kids pulled on the doll and ended up with an arm in one hand and the rest of the doll in the other. And then Carla would gaze at them intently while reciting a series of prompts: "Oh no. What happened? What did you do?" It will relieve you to know that this psychological torment lasted only 60 seconds and was followed by a period of "debriefing" in which Carla assured the child that the doll was already broken. But by then we had our videotape, and that 60-second period was revealing! Children around the age of 3 years old (those who had no false-belief understanding) showed very little shame or remorse. The same was true of the kids who were around the age of 4 (those who definitely had false-belief understanding). They might simply claim that the doll was a crappy toy. But those kids who were just getting the hang of false-belief understanding (around 3½ years old) did indeed show shame reactions. They hunched down in their chairs, averted their gaze, held their arms in front of their faces, or said how sorry they were.

The point of the experiment, and the point of this section, is that the child's understanding that other people have independent minds, with their own thoughts and opinions, allows more than just mature perspective-taking. It promotes a new anxiety that people may think badly of one another—an anxiety that reflects self-consciousness, embarrassment, and even intense shame. We see this shift in emotional dynamics as a double-edged sword. Its dark side is already obvious. But its bright side is a potential springboard along the path of moral development. Unless the child can experience shame about violating other peoples' expectations, unless he can feel self-conscious enough to want to fix his behavior, he won't be motivated to conform to the norms and standards of his family. And without that leg up, he won't have the skills or the motives to acquiesce to the norms and standards of his classroom, his community, and his society. The self-consciousness that makes its debut with false-belief understanding may be a necessary, in fact crucial, aspect of children's social-moral development. But for at least a few months, while this insight is still fresh, before the child has developed skills for coping with the anxieties it promotes, the child may be particularly vulnerable to feelings of insecurity, lapses in self-confidence, and concerns about being admired, liked, or loved.

This pendulum-swing back toward sensitivity and insecurity is the occasion for a variety of emotional concerns. These include the emergence of irrational fears, such as a recurring fear of the dark, or the worry that a person (or animal!) is angry at the child for some small wrongdoing. This is an age when bad dreams and even night terrors can proliferate. It is also an age when kids become highly compulsive, needing to act out each step in a detailed ritual when putting on their clothes, going to the bathroom, or going to bed (if they haven't already). In short, anxieties seem to increase in kind and in frequency at the age of 3½ to 4 years, and while we can't be sure they are related to theory of mind, many of them do involve concerns about being seen by others as "bad." For all these reasons, the stage of Self-consciousness at 3½ to 4 years (and beyond) requires your reassurance, your comforting, your ability to read your child's mind and know what things are like from her point of view. Now is when you need to be sensitive to her anxieties, not exacerbate them. So, if your child's sleep habits still are not up to par at this stage, go easy. Don't make any fast moves. Especially moves that will leave her wondering what you *really* think. Sleep training can wait for a few more months until the novelty of false-belief understanding is past and self-confidence returns once again.

Individual Differences

We have seen that the stages of emotional development over the first 4 years of life mark new ways of interpreting the world, giving rise to new emotional responses and new capacities for controlling those responses. And we have seen how these stages describe a pendulum-swing back and forth between periods of sensitivity and periods of resilience.

Up until now, our portrayal of theory, research findings, recommendations, and cautionary notes treats children as if they were all the same. After all, the premise of our book is that children go through normative stages at predictable ages. Obviously, we could not make these predictions if we were thinking about the individual child's personality or temperament. We have to point toward the "normative" child, the average child, the common denominator. Nevertheless, both as developmentalists and as parents (and especially as parents of twins!) we are aware of how different children can be. Individual differences take many forms and result from many causes. They can be influenced by parents and siblings, by environmental features of the home and the neighborhood, by health and dietary issues, by traumatic events, and so on. But some individual differences are at least partially built into the child's nervous system, generally through the action of genes responsible for constructing brains, glands, sense organs, and all the wiring that connects them. These variations, usually referred to as *temperament*, are not always evident at birth. Sometimes a remarkably distinct temperamental feature won't show itself until the middle or end of the first year, or even later. However, temperamental differences, by definition, are built in to the child's biological makeup and so, as a rule, they do show up early in development.

Temperament refers to the biologically based differences in children that are usually evident early in development.

Yet temperamental differences are never simply "there," hatched in their final form by the child's genetic makeup. They are always shaped by experiences in the world that have an impact on a nervous system that is still developing over childhood and adolescence. It is this interaction between "nature" (genes) and "nurture" (experience) that makes temperament so difficult, complex, and fascinating to study. For example, children who are anxious or inhibited in the middle of the first year sometimes end up as anxious/inhibited adolescents and adults, but more often end up indistinguishable from their peers. The outcome seems to depend on their social experiences. And the tendency toward depression, while stamped in genes that govern brain development, only leads to depression in certain individuals. Others grow up without depression, due in large part to the nurturance and support of parents and other caregivers. So, the "finished product" of temperament comes from an ongoing spiral of influence between genes and environment. But temperamental tendencies, and their biological foundations, are clearly seen in late infancy and early childhood, and these differences greatly affect how children will respond to emotional challenges such as sleep training. In turn, the impact of such challenges on the development of temperament (or, one could say, personality) is huge. And that's why it's of utmost importance to try to tailor emotional challenges (like sleep training) to your child's temperamental vulnerabilities.

There are many ways to divide the pie of temperament, and myriad books have been written on the subject. One of the original systems for delineating temperament styles in infants and young children was developed by Alexander Thomas and Stella Chess in the 1960s and 1970s, and we'll use this system to illustrate our ideas. According to these researchers, of the children who could be classified, about two-thirds were labeled "easy" and the remainder were divided almost equally into "difficult" and "slow to warm up." The easy child adapted smoothly to new experiences, was generally happy, and had few difficulties eating or sleeping. Difficult babies were irritable, fussy, and reactive, they cried a lot, and they tended to have irregular eating and sleep habits. Babies who were slow to warm up often would withdraw from new experiences or people, and they adapted to these experiences only slowly, after repeated exposure. The first two descriptors, easy and difficult, probably bring clear images to mind for anyone who's spent time with children. Indeed, some babies seem to take challenges and novel experiences in stride, whereas others fuss and cry when they are challenged, when their expectations aren't met, or when they are tired, or hungry, or just plain moody. The former group grow into toddlers who, though rambunctious and defiant to some degree, generally end up cooperating with parents and accepting most situations. Difficult toddlers, on the other hand, can be extremely challenging. They are the ones for whom nothing seems to work, for whom every choice is intolerable, and who fight or resist many parental directives, from putting on their socks to eating what's in front of them. The final label, "slow to warm up," seems to apply to children who were more precisely described by Jerome Kagan's research in the 1980s. Kagan delineated a group of babies who would freeze or withdraw when faced with loud noises, novel sights, and new people. He described these babies as anxious or inhibited. These anxious/inhibited children generally showed a high, regular heart rate, and they would startle easily. Just as "difficult" babies' temperaments seemed to revolve around the emotion of anger, inhibited babies' predominant emotion was anxiety or fear. Then, as mentioned, a certain proportion of these babies would grow into inhibited, overly cautious teenagers and adults, a few would develop full-blown anxiety disorders, but the majority would end up just like most other children, with no real emotional problems at all.

Temperamental differences come
from a combination of genetic
foundations and experience in the world,
especially at the hands of caregivers.

There's no empirical research that has tried to identify the best match between different temperamental styles and different sleep-training approaches. But we can highlight certain emotional features of different types of temperaments that might be relevant to the decisions you make. Difficult children may be challenging in infancy, but their behavior as toddlers can be next to impossible . . . and keep your head down during entry into the third year of life. A difficult temperament can break into a set of pivotal issues around which parent and child confront each other again and again. These emotional hot spots become nearly impossible to navigate. It's the toddler's job to be defiant, at least some of the time. But when a child is defiant most of the time, life can be hell. So we would recommend dealing with as many of these issues as possible before they become entrenched battle zones. Use the developing child's sensitivity to routines, rewards, and rules to establish set ways of doing things, from eating to dressing to cleaning up messes. For every rule learned, there will be one less issue to fight about. This may be particularly important when it comes to bedtime. Difficult babies may have trouble developing regular sleep habits regardless of parents' philosophies and efforts. That's why it's probably most important to get these kids into a regular, predictable bedtime routine as early as possible—definitely before the stage of Social Negotiation. And when you do embark on sleep training with these kids, stick closely to our guidelines. You might get away with some slack with an easy kid, but for difficult kids you will need to take advantage of the optimal windows we describe in this book.

> Keeping in mind your child's unique temperament can help you make the best decision about when to try sleep training.

Anxious/inhibited children won't have difficulties in as many situations, but the situations that prove to be difficult will be of a particular sort. These kids will have the most trouble dealing with new people and with separations. And these difficulties are likely to improve on their own with age. So try to keep these challenges in check. Provide your anxious kid with extra doses of love and nurturance when out visiting others, or on holidays, and try not to compound the anxieties brought about by novelty with those arising from separation and loss. These considerations will be especially important in those stages of development marked by separation distress. So we suggest providing your anxious/inhibited child with loads of familiarity, and especially with access to his parents for protection and security, during the periods of Social Referencing and Social Negotiation. Of course separation issues will create extra challenges for sleep training. So you should definitely avoid sleep training during these two stages. Instead, shoot for the stages of greatest individual autonomy and resilience: Motor Initiative and Motor Practice. Motor Initiative might be especially well-suited for sleep training, as it comes before your child has ever experienced true separation distress. Finally, take care never to combine sleep training with prolonged parental absence or the presence of unfamiliar adults. Don't even think about babysitters until after sleep training has settled into a stable and predictable habit.

Finally, if your child is best described as easy, relax! You're going to have the easiest time with most emotional challenges, sleep training included. In fact, you might get away with deviating from our prescribed sequence of optimal windows. We don't advise too much deviation, but if uncontrollable events like returning to work, moving house, or dealing with another child make it difficult to stick with our stage-by-stage schedule, you'll still have a reasonable shot at successful sleep training during nonoptimal periods. And less serious consequences if things don't work out.

Now, on to the nuts and bolts of getting your child to sleep through the night and nap regularly during the day. The following chapters get into the practical matters of sleep training in greater detail than was possible in Chapter 3, and in a format designed for easy reference and on-the-spot guidance. But the groundwork has been laid; the developmental knowledge is yours. And that knowledge makes you as much an expert as anyone in facing the challenges of parenting—not only in the realm of sleep training but also in many other areas.

4

Windows of Opportunity

When to Sleep Train and When to Wait

YOU MAY BELIEVE IN TEACHING YOUR CHILD to learn to sleep on her own by letting her "cry it out" for as long as it takes, or picking her up every time she cries and rocking her back to sleep with gentle words, or patting her quietly in her crib until she falls asleep, or letting her cry for brief periods before coming back in to reassure her. We firmly believe that most methods of sleep training that have been written about are legitimate and can lead to excellent results for both the child and family. But we also believe that *all* sleep-training methods have the potential to fail, creating excessive distress for the child and parent, and leading to poor sleep habits that can last throughout a child's life. From our perspective, the likelihood that your child will easily learn to sleep on her own has less to do with the precise technique you choose than with *when* you apply it.

This chapter provides a complete guide to the stages that are problematic for getting your child to sleep and those that make it relatively easy. In particular, we'll warn you against sleep training during the periods when young children are most vulnerable to separation distress; insecurities regarding your whereabouts or affections; feelings of shame, jealousy, or exclusion; and other interpersonal challenges. No matter how determined and conscientious you are, and no matter how good the advice you're following, you should try to avoid these stages when you're introducing this new set of demands. And they *are* demands. You are requiring your child to revamp one of the most basic habits in the human repertoire: the way he falls asleep. And falling asleep usually requires being left alone. This is a big deal in your child's life! We think that sleep training does far more good than harm in most households, but it is still a challenge for both child and parent. And because it is difficult, your child should be at his best when you begin sleep training. This chapter details when he is likely to be at his best and his worst—at least when it comes to saying good night.

> Because it is challenging and difficult,
> your child should be at her best
> when you begin sleep training.

Take a look at Figure 3 on pages 130 to 131. It gives you a quick summary of the ages and stages that are best- and worst-suited for sleep training. If your child's age falls in any of the gray zones, wait until she's past that stage. If it falls in one of the white zones, then go for it! The laws of child development are on your side. It's about time that you and your child got the best night's sleep you possibly can. And we hope it will reassure you to know that if you're ready to start sleep training, in all likelihood so is your child . . . as long as you stick to the easy stages. What we also spell out in this chapter are some of the specific issues to attend to when sleep training at the worst and best stages. Six months and 3 years are both appropriate ages to begin sleep training. But you are dealing with a different animal at each age, so there are different goals, concerns, potential pitfalls, trade-offs, and specific tricks to consider for each.

> There are certain ages and stages
> during which the laws of development
> are on your side and sleep training
> can be a breeze.

Of course, children really are different, and our guidelines are in no way meant to be taken as absolute. Because of an easy temperament, a particular family structure, or other fortunate circumstances, your child might defy our schedule and fall asleep very nicely in the periods we deem difficult. But overall, if you're flexible about when to start sleep training, and if your child is what you'd call "typical," you should try to target your efforts to the next easy period.

Also, we'd like to let you in on a well-kept secret: most parents have to sleep train their children more than once. Children get sick, they get moved from their crib to "big boy beds," they go on family vacations during which routines change, siblings are born, and so on. Many factors can disrupt hard-won sleep skills, and then you're stuck teaching these skills again, in an entirely different developmental window. So even if you've used this book

Figure 3. Ages and Stages for Avoiding or Implementing Sleep Training

Approximate Age	Emotional Stage	Reasons to Avoid Sleep Training	Reasons to Start Sleep Training
0–2½ months	1: Basic Regulation	• basic biological rhythms, including day–night differentiation, need to develop without interference	
2½–4 months	2: Interpersonal Attention		• babies now have a regular day–night cycle, which can be adjusted • babies are more sociable but show no separation distress
4–5½ months	3: Interpersonal Expectancy	• babies expect their actions to produce some response from parents • big changes include growing autonomy and a new sense of an interpersonal bond	
5½–7½ months	4: Motor Initiative		• this is a very robust stage, when babies are more interested in grasping objects and moving their bodies than tracking caregivers' whereabouts
8–11 months	5: Social Referencing	• object permanence, social referencing, and search for absent people make separations particularly difficult • babies constantly test parents' availability	
12–16 months	6: Motor Practice		• upright locomotion and delight in the physical world reduce dependency • babies show improved physical coordination • babbling and proto-speech can replace absent parent

Age	Stage	Description
17–21 months	7: Social Negotiation	• toddlers gain an understanding of others' goals and complementary roles • toddlers now see relationships as social and try to establish both security and independence • intense needs for attention, closeness, and reassurance produce a peak in separation distress
22–27 months	8: Social Stabilization	• many babies have established secure feelings and are more open to adjustments in their social habits • toddlers now wish to please others and adapt to rules
28 months–3 years	9: Social Comparison	• this is a highly unpredictable period • along with social manipulation, real jealousy emerges and induces shame and self-doubt • stubbornness and defiance may increase
3–3½ years	10: Family Membership	• children now understand their role in the family • rules and feelings come together in newfound diplomacy • close connections with stuffed animals and dolls are comforting
3½–4 years	11: Self-consciousness	• children begin to understand that others have minds of their own • many children express insecurity based on fears of being seen as "bad" • self-consciousness and more intense shame reactions develop

once to identify the best upcoming age to sleep train, you may want to keep your copy handy, in case a sleep setback requires you to find another optimal window for retraining your child.

Stage 1
Basic Regulation: 0 to 2½ months

As detailed in Chapter 3, this is a time in which the baby's sensory controls, motor capacities, and key physiological functions emerge and begin to stabilize. A child's abilities to pay attention, sustain or shift interest, drink, digest, and eliminate, are turned on and coordinated. As a result, the baby can soon swivel his gaze around to follow an object of interest, or hold on to a toy or your finger for minutes at a time, or lie still and suck on the breast or bottle until satisfied. Most important, this is an age when the baby's states—alert attention, quiet wakefulness, and sleep—become practiced and differentiated from each other, creating a predictable cycle of daily rhythms. And these rhythms gradually become synchronized with the day-and-night cycle of our planet, so that, starting around 6 weeks, babies sleep more at night and less in the day. And, as they develop, these rhythms will also become synchronized with the caregivers' rhythms and the household routines that underlie them. As we discussed in Chapter 3, you can tell that the Basic Regulation period has been successfully completed when your baby can shift states smoothly and easily and when you and your baby begin to work together as a team, especially with respect to feeding, playing, and—to at least some degree—sleeping. You will also notice a rapid increase in face-to-face gazing, more smiling and other expressions of pleasure, and a general decrease in fussiness at the end of this stage. Babies learn, by about 2½ to 3 months, that they are part of a complex but exciting world of cycles both inside and outside their bodies.

Sleep training prior to 2½ to 3 months is not a good idea. There is too much going on. The synchronization of brain and bodily systems, the establishment of cycles for eating and sleeping, the coordination of these cycles with the outside world—all need time to develop and stabilize. The sheer number of biological and psychological systems getting wired up, and the rapid rate at which they are becoming connected with one another, staggers the imagination. Babies are extremely complicated "machines" whose functioning gets perfected in a series of "test drives" in a complicated world. The fact that habits and skills develop out of this matrix of change is remarkable in itself. A lot of biological events, including cascades of changes in neural pathways and organ systems, unfold with uncanny precision, almost as if there were a master schedule posted somewhere and your baby were diligently following it. Scientists still do not know exactly how this cascade of changes progresses so effectively. But what we do know, as child psychologists, is that it's better not to mess with it! To attempt sleep training before your baby does the majority of her sleeping at night would be to miss a massive biological boost. We suggest letting natural biological processes do their work before you begin adjusting the fine points. Even after day–night differentiation is complete, we advise parents to let the rapid changes of this period taper off, resulting in a stable and robust little organism who fits well and feels secure in the world of sensations, movements, and human interactions in which she'll spend the rest of her life.

Sleep training during the period of Basic Regulation may simply be ineffective. It may be difficult or impossible to establish desirable sleep habits before sleeping at night becomes routine. But it could also confuse your baby's evolving capacity to synchronize his interest, excitement levels, perception, and communication. Imagine that your baby is just learning to smile at you and to expect a smile in return. This reciprocal smiling sets off an episode of communication that is designed to *increase arousal*, because arousal is part of pleasure. And now imagine that this smiling takes place just as you are turning out the lights and leaving the room, a necessary step in most sleep-training protocols. Now your aroused, excited baby, instead of receiving the ongoing communication he expects, is faced with the prospect of lying still and going to sleep. This might simply not work, as mentioned above. But it's quite possible that after a few such scenarios, your baby will become confused as to what to expect when mutual smiling or gazing take place. *Maybe the smiling means "game over." Maybe I should disengage rather than engage when Mom and I make eye contact.* This sort of interpersonal confusion could result from mixed signals, as the baby sees it, at this vulnerable age. Better to wait until the interpersonal routines of smiling and gazing become solid habits. As they solidify, security and trust will solidify as well, making the ordeal of sleep training less of a challenge to your baby's sense of himself, his sense of you, and his sense of your relationship.

Is there anything you can do about the seemingly chaotic sleep schedule of your newborn? Our answer is best summarized in John Lennon's song "Whatever Gets You Through the Night." Use a swing, a bouncy chair, tuck your baby in the crook of your neck, lay her across your chest, rock her in a chair, a glider, or a hammock, bounce her in a sling or a baby carrier, throw her in a car seat on top of the dryer, in the backseat of a car, or in the stroller. Anything you do, we guarantee you, you can undo with proper sleep training at a later stage of development. This is not the time to stress out about "creating bad habits." What you're creating is a tight bond with a rapidly developing little organism that needs your warmth, flexibility, and consistency. During this early newborn stage, whatever gets you (and your baby) through the night is just fine.

Stage 2
Interpersonal Attention: 2½ to 4 months
We described this stage as the period when Basic Regulation finally consolidates, when babies' physiological, sensory, motor, and emotional capacities have started to become coordinated and are now working in sync with each other. It's an age when the baby's sleep habits start to regularize, with or without your intervention, when day–night cycles start to materialize, and it's an age when mother's and baby's behaviors become coordinated. Now, mutual gazing, smiling, cooing, hugging, nursing, holding, and rocking all begin to establish their own rhythms, because you and your baby have become real partners in the physical management of his bodily routines. Unexplained distress is on

the wane, social smiles begin to flourish, your baby is looking "at" you, with real interest, excitement, and the beginnings of love.

Before this time, sleep training was not advisable, because your baby's sleep–wake cycles were too disjointed, as were the other routines of his existence. He just couldn't get it together yet. But now, before a new stage of cognitive development stirs up the pot again, you are in a period of relative stability and resilience. Sleep training is not likely to interfere with the laying down of fundamental routines. But are you ready? Is this the right time for you? Many parents feel that 2½ to 4 months is still too early. Even though bodily routines have become coordinated, the baby is far from "finished." In particular, the mother–infant relationship is now the source of a whole lot of pleasure for both of you. Such smiles! Such long, penetrating gazes! And this kid is getting cute! He used to look like a little alien, too round in some facial features, too pointed in others. You wondered whether his ears would ever fit his head. And look at him now! Especially in those snazzy overalls. He is becoming a good-looking kid (perhaps a little more in your eyes than anyone else's). As mothers watch their babies "become human," sleeping more at night than in the day, crying less, smiling more, and looking rather handsome when out on the town, they often feel that development is proceeding well on its own. So why mess with it? Besides, when babies wake up at night prior to 4 months or so, it's usually because they're hungry. So how much sleep training is appropriate? According to this line of thought, now is not the right time to interfere. Let nature take its course.

Although 2½ to 4 months is too early
for some parents to sleep train,
it is the first window of opportunity
for those at their wits' end.

And you are probably getting more sleep at night than you have since day one, even without any consistent attempts to mold your baby's sleep habits.

MICHAEL AND MEREDITH'S STORY

Let Sleeping Babes Lie

Things have taken a turn for the better, suddenly, at 3 months. Oliver is sleeping 5 hours at a stretch at night. He sleeps from 7 p.m. to 1 a.m., gets fed, and then sleeps until 4 or 5 a.m., when he's hungry once again. "Not bad," says Michael. "Fantastic," says Meredith. "Until just before 3 months, Oliver woke up every 2 to 3 hours throughout the night. But now he seems to be training himself. We'd like to see how far he gets, how much more progress he makes on his own, before we put him on a schedule. There is ample opportunity to introduce sleep training when Oliver hits 6 months. Why not see how he does on his own right now?"

Many parents feel the same as Michael and Meredith. And many parents simply can't bring themselves to stop responding to their child's cries at night. There are too many questions they simply can't answer. Why is he awake now? Is he still hungry? Does he have gas? Is he lonely? Did he nap too long earlier? Maybe he just needs a cuddle . . . he's still so, so small. Maybe it's a growth spurt and he's hungry more often. With all these explanations still making sense, some parents feel it is just too early to begin sleep training.

Other parents feel that the sooner you start sleep training, the better. Let's get this over with. Indeed, why not do it at an age when there will be no traumatic memories laid down, an age before babies can even remember that their mother was just here and now she's gone, an age when babies respond to Mom's presence with great pleasure but seem almost indifferent to her absence? They usually don't cry when Mom leaves the room, so why not take advantage of this natural oasis and put it to some use? This thinking makes a lot of sense as well. There is no good reason not to try sleep training at this age if your intuition says "go!" and your baby responds favorably. So what are the things to think about if you do embark on sleep training now?

As always, be aware of the cost-benefit ratio that comes with sleep training. Of course there are vast differences in how you'll measure the "costs," depending on the method you use and the age at which you try it. But at 2½ to 4 months, outright distress of more than a few minutes is an obvious cost. How long does your baby cry when falling asleep *without* the usual props, whether the breast or bottle, holding, rocking, or any other form of ongoing physical contact? You may expect some distress, again depending on your method, but how much is too much? At this tender age, distress quickly takes over the infant's whole body and becomes increasingly difficult to regulate over a period of several minutes. Babies' skills at regulating their emotions just don't go far without the fundamental awareness that actions lead to outcomes. The limbs become rigid, breathing becomes forced and difficult, crying becomes shrill and ghastly, and the face turns into a rictus of seeming pain, even though we have no reason to think that the baby really is in physical pain of any kind. If this level of distress ensues when you start sleep training, and if it takes over and lasts for 5 or 10 minutes, that may be more than enough. Young babies have a hard time recovering from this pattern of intense distress, and past a certain threshold they may continue to cry until exhaustion sets in. This may be a signal that now is not the right time.

There is no rule to help you through these decisions. If you've been getting up every hour or two throughout the night to feed, rock, or otherwise soothe your baby, then you are probably willing to keep trying for a few days, despite periods of intense distress, and see if your sleep-training method "takes." We don't blame you. In fact we would cheer you on! Going through the next few months of your life in a state of utter exhaustion is not in anybody's best interests. Try to get past the distress by making minor adjustments to the method you've applied. Have yourself a sizable glass or two of wine if the crying is killing you. Think about how long you want to try—in advance!—before you decide whether your method is working. At this age, you should know within 5 days to a week if your baby is adjusting to the new routines. If intense distress continues to be a regular part of bedtime after a week, you'd best consider some alternatives. But if, like Meredith and Michael, sleep habits were already beginning to improve nicely, then the cost of intense distress, for even a few days, may be more than you should pay. You may decide instead to wait until the next window of opportunity—5½ to 7½ months.

There are other trade-offs to consider. Given the amount of distress caused by sleep training, how many extra hours of sleep are you buying? If, after a long bout of crying, your baby finally does go to sleep, but then wakes up again 45 minutes later, the cost is not worth the benefit. The trauma for you and your baby isn't paying for itself in much rest for either of you. And you're getting a message here that can't be ignored. If sleep training is only gaining you a short respite, then your baby is probably waking up for good reasons. Most likely, he's hungry. He may also be wet, or uncomfortable, but those factors are easily corrected. If nothing else seems to be wrong, the most obvious reason for frequent wakings at this age is hunger. And if your baby simply needs to feed more often than you might have hoped, or more often than your best friend's baby, there may be nothing you can do about it. So save yourself and your child the trouble and go with his rhythms for now. You've lasted this long: you can last a little longer. And her digestive system is continuing to mature. She will not need to feed every 3 hours several months from now. You may be up against a whole lot less if you delay sleep training until then.

Parents will often choose sleep training at the young age of 2½ to 4 months because there is a real need to do so. You may have to go back to work, and functioning on 3 to 4 hours of sleep is impossible after a few days. If you are spending much of your night feeding, rocking, and soothing your child, or if she is still waking every hour or two, then you are a basket case. You're exhausted. Your mood is seriously affected and you can't be the parent you envisioned for yourself. You may have hit "rock bottom" and become diagnosably anxious or depressed. If this sounds familiar, we recommend you try your best to make sleep training work. Now, not later. This isn't selfish of you! Your baby will feel a lot better if she is well rested. And so will you: you need your sleep. If you're walking into walls, leaving the stove on, just about to be fired, or screaming at your husband or other children, then it's time to make a change, for everyone's sake, and it's worth the hard work of sleep training.

This first window for sleep training isn't everyone's cup of tea, and its success will depend in large part on your baby's temperament, her baseline fussiness and sensitivity to noise and other intrusions, and her digestive maturity—how long she can last with a stomach full of milk. If you feel like trying sleep training at this age, then go for it! Good luck. Do your best. If it doesn't work, you only have a few more months to wait until the next window of opportunity.

Stage 3
Interpersonal Expectancy: 4 to 5½ months

If you've waited until now, wait a little longer. The period of 4 to 5½ months is not recommended for sleep training for several reasons. As discussed in Chapter 2, the age of 4 months is the beginning of a major stage transition in cognitive development.

Babies are now beginning to coordinate simple actions, like reaching and grasping, into operations that have a deliberate impact on the world. Now your baby can actually reach what he's aiming for, put it in his mouth, and explore it. That means that objects are accessible, reachable, touchable, and mouthable. But more than that, babies at this age are beginning to develop motor *expectancies*. When they reach, they expect what they reach for to be there. Having this prediction confirmed time after time gives them a sense that their actions are causing a particular effect. Piaget termed this level of cause–effect thinking "magico-phenomenalistic causality," which just means that the baby has a kind of magical expectation that his actions will produce desirable effects. With respect to people, these growing expectations are the key to gratifying exchanges of smiles and gestures. As outlined in Chapter 3, babies will now make a noise in order to elicit a smile from the caregiver. In other words, this is a time for building up sequences of back-and-forth communication and play. A time when attention to other people is not just a static state of awestruck delight, but a state of active expectancy, when every noise, every gesture, is offered in order to get a response from the other person. That response means everything.

So why not sleep train at this age? Like the development of Basic Regulation at birth to 2½ months, a set of critical abilities is coming together at just this point in the baby's life. In this case it is a set of motor skills connected to perceptual expectancies—expectancies about the other person's response—all of which result in the establishment of interpersonal habits of intentional, heartfelt communication. It is best not to rock the boat at this time, not to perturb these budding abilities until they have become well practiced and stabilized. In other words, it is important not to disturb the baby's new set of interpersonal goals and skills until they've really begun to solidify—until the baby gains some confidence that other people really do act the way he expects them to.

In Chapter 3 we explained that this set of cognitive and emotional changes results in a new kind of bond between the infant and caregiver. We talked about the development of the baby's new sense of self—a self that feels independent and autonomous. We went on to show that this sense of self combines with a sense of the other person as a playmate, a caring respondent to the baby's bids for action and connection. Back-and-forth interaction, while very new at this age, is an important kind of cement for binding your baby's new sense of self with his sense of parents who are responsive, predictable, and reliable. Now imagine that you have just discovered that there are magical things you can do with the world of objects: reach out and grab things and bring them close to you. And at the same time you are finding that those big humans who hold you and smile at you are also responding to your signals, doing what you want them to do. Not only can you play with them using your new skills, maintaining that sense of control and predictability, but also you can get that special feeling of warmth and love that comes only from humans. And then, suddenly one evening, just when you thought you were playing together, the big humans go away. You reach out and they're not there. You wait for a voice, a tickle, or a laugh, and it doesn't come. This could be confusing or even disturbing. It could produce immediate frustration as well as more long-lasting disappointment. And, over repeated occasions, such feelings might contribute to a sense of irritation or insecurity, as expressed by increasingly intense distress reactions (something over which you have no control).

> Sleep training between 4 and 5½ months can produce frustration and confusion, because your baby needs you to be her playmate.

Here is one woman's account of sleep training at 4 months. She had twins to contend with, so her challenges were considerably greater than those of many parents.

NATALIE'S STORY

Trial by Crier

The baby was 4½ months when we went for it. We were planning on waiting until 5 or even 6 months, but it had gotten *so* bad: we were rocking (bouncing on a ball, actually) and soothing him to sleep for literally hours every night— and for naps too! The straw that broke the camel's back was the afternoon that I had soothed my son for an hour and a half, only to find that the second I lay him down he would wake up and scream again to be held. I couldn't take it

anymore. I told him, "I love you, little fella. You can do this."
And I put him down and that was it. The crying began. We
were in Ferberizing hell for 4 weeks (and I have the Cry Chart
to prove it). It involved hours and hours of crying and wailing.

There is also a more general reason to avoid sleep training at
this age. Four to 5 months is the cusp of a major shift in development. The changes taking place at this time are massive: your
baby is transforming from a relatively passive creature, busy perceiving the world, into an active being with clear intentions, ready
to reach out and engage with anything and anyone. The philosophy underlying our approach is to avoid compounding stressful
periods with the additional stress of sleep training. Let your baby
reestablish some predictability, in her actions, her emotional
reactions, and her expectations regarding your responses. Then,
once these changes settle down, an ideal window for sleep training presents itself again, at about 5½ to 7½ months.

Stage 4
Motor Initiative: 5½ to 7½ months

This stage of development is often the optimal window for sleep
training. The changes put in motion by a massive shift in cognitive development (the onset of Actions & Outcomes at 4 to 5
months) have now begun to stabilize. Your baby continues to
develop new talents and capacities, but they are refinements
of skills he's already achieved, and they generally involve the
nonhuman world of toys and other objects. At the same time,
he is able to be left alone for longer and longer periods. He

may have begun to sit up by himself by now, in which case it's even easier for him to amuse himself without your intervention, because he can reach for what he wants in almost any direction. But if not, then he can lie on his back or his belly, either pulling at a mobile over his head or reaching for new and interesting things to put in his mouth. He is very interested in this world of *things.* He knows you're around. He doesn't always know exactly where, but he senses that he is not alone. He is a relatively secure little fellow, especially compared to the more volatile baby of 2 months ago. And, most important, he has not yet learned how to search for vanished objects—or vanished parents! Before 8 to 9 months, he can't hold enough information in working memory to keep track of whatever or whoever has disappeared while manipulating the physical world to get it (or her) back. That means that the parent who leaves the room is usually disregarded within a few moments. We know. It seems odd. Infants at this age don't really think you've gone for good. It's more like they can't be bothered trying to get you back. It's too difficult. They don't know how. They figure you'll show up whenever you show up. And, as a result, they do not experience separation distress.

For most sleep-training approaches, some kind of physical separation takes place before your baby falls asleep. Even if you use techniques that involve staying with your child until after he falls asleep, waking up to your absence may still be traumatic. If your child is old enough to be sensitive to these issues, then it doesn't take long for that absence to become associated with bedtime itself. Bedtime still means that mom and dad are gone. In both of these kinds of scenarios, separation distress, or separation anxiety, is a big deal. And if you haven't watched a child go through the pangs of this particular form of distress, take our word for it: it is heart-wrenching. A child who is waiting for her mom to return, who knows she's out there, who wishes with all her might that she'd come back, will escalate from anxious whining to a spiral of distress, often wailing, shouting, and crying, sometimes for long periods, up to an hour or more, before sheer exhaustion sets in. Separation distress is one of the most intense (normal) traumas for the infant, and if you can avoid it, then you're ahead of the game.

For that reason alone, sleep training prior to 8 months is a good idea for many families. How fortunate you are that your baby is not at an age where separations are meaningful and distressing. You can leave the room without triggering that spiral of painful feelings. You can say good night, walk out that door, and leave behind an infant who is fairly content. What you'll hear, if sleep training is going well and instead of the wailing you might have expected, are the contented sounds of a baby sucking on his fist or soother, or the rustling of sheets as he creeps about from one edge of the crib to the other, or the surprising coos and gurgles of a child whose voice box is more entertaining than any radio station, emitting as it does the most amazing of sounds. This infant is generally more interested in interacting with the world of things than the world of people, and people can come and go without eliciting much concern.

Sleep training before 8 to 9 months
means you generally don't have to deal
with intense separation distress.

In a nutshell, the stage of Motor Initiative is such a good time for sleep training because you have at your disposal a well-regulated baby, whose physiological and psychological states are relatively well organized, and whose states shift from one to the next easily and smoothly, who is relatively autonomous, who is excited and delighted by the world of sights and sounds and especially by the capacity to manipulate objects, to reach for them, grasp them, and suck on them. You have, in a word, a little creature who enjoys living in the world, who belongs in the world, and who is not particularly focused on you to get her through the day. Or night. And, as a bonus, this little creature is immune to separation distress. No matter how interested she may be in watching you come and go, no matter how brightly she smiles at you when you bounce her or talk with her, she quickly goes back to her own activities when you've left the room. Sleep train any earlier and your baby is less regulated, more raw, less stable. Sleep train any later and your baby will surely feel the pangs of separation distress to at least some degree. In fact, sleep training at this age comes before any long-term habits have built up. Your baby is still a newcomer in the world, and for that simple reason much more malleable than she will be later on.

At this age, sleep training can happen so quickly that it's over and done with while you thought you were still warming up. But every family forges its own path. Here's Julie's account of what it was like to retrain her twin infants after the disastrous experience of trying to get them to sleep at 4½ months.

JULIE'S STORY
Together at Last

Our twins were always separated for sleep training, from day one. We tried to put them back into the same room at around 4½ months, but all hell broke loose. Neither slept well, and we just gave up. Then, at about 6½ months, we tried again to put them in one room to sleep. My husband and I wanted our own room back to ourselves. We were scared to death to put them back together again. But lo and behold, it was smooth like buttah! Sara moved back into her crib, and she and her brother now sleep in their own room— which Mommy and Daddy *love*. They don't wake each other. It's quite amazing, really.

Sleep training in the stage of Motor Initiative can thus be pretty seamless. Indeed, "like buttah." But there are a few things to watch out for. Many parents choose to swaddle their babies during the first 6 months or so. You know those days are over when, no matter how clever you've become at tying, folding, and knotting the swaddling blanket, your baby is now a little Houdini who can miraculously escape. All he has to do is get one arm out, which is possible because he's figured out how to loosen the blanket by wiggling his bottom in a certain way, and then it's a lost cause. Knowing that your swaddling days are numbered, you'll want to orchestrate sleep training in a thoughtful way so that the two changes don't work against each other. Should you complete sleep training first, then remove the swaddling blanket and replace it with some very warm pyjamas once he's sleeping through the night? Or should you phase out swaddling and phase in sleep training at the same time? There are no formulaic answers to these questions. But like many of the caretaking decisions you're going to make, this one will require your intelligence, creativity, and common sense.

Another issue interwoven with sleep training at this age will inevitably be night feeding. Are you going to go for broke? Are you going to try for 8, 10, even 12 hours of peace? There's no doubt that the 6- to 7-month-old baby can sleep for that long . . . *if* she doesn't wake up starving in the meantime. Think about how to shake your baby loose from that 2 a.m. feeding in order to maximize the chances for a full night's sleep. Do you want to wean her from the breast? That isn't a prerequisite for getting 12 hours of sleep, but it sure can help. Do you want to replace the breast with the bottle a few times a day? Or only at night? In advance of sleep training, so that the new habits have had a chance to take? You're going to have to think about the steps involved. Some mothers gradually reduce the amount of milk they give their baby for the nighttime feeding, so that she gets used to acquiring most of her calories during the day. There is also a useful little trick: adding more and more water to the midnight bottle, eventually reducing the proportion of milk to nothing, so that the baby can drop that feeding without losing anything in the way of nutrition. The timing, amount, and type of solid foods, and the age at which they're introduced, may also have a major impact on nighttime hunger. These are all things to consider when you go for a cry-free night during the stage of Motor Initiative.

Other issues will depend on the configuration of your house, on other family members, and especially on other children. Your baby is now old enough to be alert to what's going on around him, and the kind and amount of nighttime noise can make or break sleep training at this age. Once his new sleep habits have begun to solidify, you can breathe a little easier, and other family members may be able to lower themselves from their tiptoes. You might want to use a fan—as a white-noise generator—until then. Whatever the considerations, the strategies, the tricks, trials, tribulations, and errors you face during this period, we predict that sleep training from 5½ to 7½ months will be easier than at any other stage.

Stage 5
Social Referencing: 8 to 11 months

There are all kinds of reasons why you may have chosen to wait it out this long. Perhaps you've had your baby sleep next to you in a family bed, or she still required two night feedings—some babies are simply hungrier than others. Whatever your reasons, you may now decide it's time. Your baby is 8 to 9 months old, she is clearly becoming more of her own person, and you are tired of having playtime between 2 and 4 a.m. Or maybe you have to go back to work and you simply can't afford the prolonged bedtime rituals or the sleep loss that goes with them. *Stop in your tracks!* The period of 8 to 11 months is one of the worst times to begin sleep training. If you've waited this long, we suggest that you wait a few more months, until the next window of opportunity, beginning around 12 months.

We have heard many stories from parents who tried to commence sleep training at 8 to 9 months, and they are almost always negative. In fact, we think this is the age that is most likely to turn a parent off sleep training. After repeated failures at this stage of your baby's life, you may want to give up on sleep training forever! Here's what some parents have said about trying to teach their children to sleep at 8 to 9 months of age.

Jenny was in the habit of rocking her baby girl to sleep every night. Then she and her husband started letting her "cry it out" at bedtime and naps at the age of 9 months. They let their daughter watch a quiet video . . .

JENNY'S STORY
Basket Case Baby

. . . and then we put her into the crib, said good night, and walked out the door. The problem was that after several weeks the baby was still getting pretty hysterical. She would cry somewhere between 15 and 45 minutes, nonstop, and showed no change over time. In fact, by the end of this period, she was still a basket case, just like she was on day one. I am beginning to feel cruel, but she really has to learn how to go to sleep on her own!

We included the following quotation from Karen in Chapter 1, but it's such a common example of what can happen at this age that we decided to include it again.

KAREN'S STORY
Bye-Bye Rock-a-Bye

Okay, I will admit I have always rocked my boy to sleep. Of course, now I am paying dearly for it! He's almost 9 months old and cannot go to sleep on his own. I want to let him cry it out, but he spits up a lot. . . . I can't go in while he's crying because that will just make him more hysterical. He also gets super clingy the day after I try to get him to cry himself to sleep. When I do it, he never lets me put him down the next day!

We feel for Jenny, Karen, and other parents like them. They're all great moms trying their best to do what's right for their kids. They've done nothing wrong, there's nothing to feel guilty about, and there's probably nothing they can do about their child's sleep problems during this stage. Our advice: if you've waited this long, wait a little longer. Time is probably the only thing that will make things better.

Why is the 8 to 11 month period so difficult for sleep training? The problem stems largely from the cognitive milestones of the Point & Click stage described in Chapter 2: the baby's ability to link one coordination with a second coordination, allowing for joint attention, social referencing, and, most important, the search for hidden objects. As discussed in Chapter 3, this cognitive advance has profound implications for emotional development. This is the age when nearly all babies start to use double coordinations to get others to help them meet their needs, to point, to read cues, to engage with others in mutual goals, and to search for people who have disappeared from view. The ability to search for vanished objects and people plays a critical role in babies' emotional reactions to separations at this age, so let's examine this issue in some depth.

Figure 4. Level of Separation Distress, from 0 to 20 Months

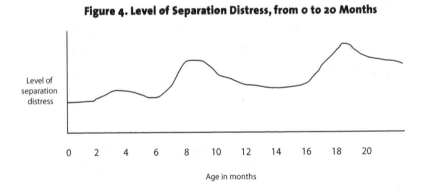

By 6 or 7 months, babies will certainly be aware that a toy or a person has disappeared from view, and they may gaze intently at the place where the disappearance occurred. But only for a few moments. Then their gaze wanders about the room, and before long they forget about the vanished object completely. This is one of the most surprising and counterintuitive features of mid-infancy. Hide a treasured toy under a mat—right in front of the baby's eyes—and your 7-month-old will invariably fail to lift the mat to find it. It's as if the vanished object has disappeared from existence. Do it over and over, showing the baby that you are hiding the toy he wants so much under the mat right in front of his face, and he will repeatedly look around, clueless, when the toy is hidden. Try it for yourself. (Go ahead, the rest of this chapter can wait. . . .)

This "cluelessness" lifts between 8 and 9 months. Due to the changes in information processing described in Chapter 2, 8- to 9-month-olds become capable of keeping the vanished object in mind while they lift whatever it is that's covered it. Now they know that a vanished object can be retrieved. And that means that a vanished parent can be retrieved too. At 7 months, if you walked out the door and didn't come back, there's a good chance your baby stopped looking for you in less than a minute. But if you try the same disappearing act 2 to 3 months later, your baby will almost certainly do everything in her power to get you back. She will not forget that you're out there. If she wants you, she will yell, scream, and cry in frustration, knowing that you are accessible and yet stubbornly refusing to reappear.

For your 9-month-old, you are no longer out of sight, out of mind.

The obsession with vanishing parents coincides with a sharp increase in separation distress, as we noted in Chapter 3. In Figure 4 on page 154, you will see a clear peak in separation distress at exactly 9 months. The rise in separation distress is precisely because separations now *mean* something to your baby.

When you separate, you are frustrating your baby's immediate attempts to get you back! That may not be how you see it, but that's how your baby sees it. No wonder he's distressed! So the point here is simple: a time when separations are most frustrating, upsetting, and even traumatic for your baby is not the right time to initiate sleep training. Sleep training inevitably involves leaving your baby alone. For the 8- to 11-month-old, this may be the most intense frustration imaginable.

> Separation anxiety begins around
> 8 to 9 months, making this stage
> one of the worst times to sleep train.

We refer to the 8 to 11 month stage as Social Referencing, and this label corresponds to a host of changes in the interpersonal domain—changes that don't lend themselves to sleep training. We covered the theory in Chapter 3, but to refresh your memory, here is a list of the changes in interpersonal cognition that are commonly observed at this age:

- intentional efforts to get parents to help the baby achieve goals
- pointing so that parents will look at a specific object
- following others' pointing, to look at a specific object
- the tendency to look to parents for emotional cues (social referencing)
- the tendency to share perceptions of the world with adults (joint attention)

- the first glimmer of understanding that other people have their own intentions
- an obsession to search for parents who have suddenly disappeared

As a result of the same cognitive advance that gives rise to separation reactions, babies now see their caregivers in a new way. They see you as someone with whom to share their experiences, someone who gives meaning to their experiences, someone with a will or intention of your own but whose intentions can be harnessed in order to fulfill their own needs. They see you as someone who needs to be checked to make sure you're ready to swoop down and help them when they need it. Joint attention means that you see things the same way they do. In other words, the parent who is so avidly sought when she leaves the room is not the same parent she was a few months ago. She is now a social partner, and that partnership can be maintained only by demands and pleas for connection and cooperation. The baby has only his own voice, his own demands, to hold on to the bonds of attention and meaning that have so recently sprung up.

So what happens when you leave the room? First, your baby will want to understand the meaning of your departure by checking with you. That's social referencing. That's joint attention. But if you don't come back into the room, she can't pick up any cues. Her demands are now likely to escalate rapidly in the form of calling out for you. Second, your baby will try to figure out where you are. Are you just outside the door? Are you in the next room? By this age, your baby has a primitive map of the house in her mind, and efforts to get you back require, first and foremost, assessing your whereabouts. Third, and perhaps most disturbing, your baby really wants to know if you intend to come when she calls you. This is a key aspect of her attempts to understand and think about your goals, not just your actions. Your baby is trying to use her new cognitive tools to maintain a new kind of relationship with you, based on a shared mental and emotional world. Most sleep-training methods require you to withdraw at least a small amount of attention and many want you to ignore your baby's calls, at least for some period of time, before going back into the room. But this ignoring explains precisely why Jenny's baby is a "basket case," and Karen's son is so "clingy" the next day. By ignoring the 9-month-old's calls to you, you are giving the message that you *aren't* on the same page, you are *not* sharing the same perceptions and feelings, your intentions *aren't* accessible, and you simply *aren't* available when she needs you. That message triggers not only distress and even desperation in the moment but also excessive neediness and insecurity in the days and nights to follow. Only when this vulnerability dies down does your baby become confident that you will respond to her needs in a way that's predictable and comforting, and only then is sleep training likely to lose these traumatic overtones. For most babies, this means waiting until 11 to 12 months.

Stage 6
Motor Practice: 12 to 16 months

It turns out that the stage of Motor Practice is a good time for sleep training for many infants—second only to Motor Initiative.

And that's because you are dealing with an infant who has many of the same qualities.

A 12- to 16-month-old child is in another emotionally stable period that is perfect for teaching him good sleep habits.

In both these stages, the child is taken with his own physical command of the world of inanimate objects. The younger infant manipulated them with his hands, while the older infant is up on his feet, cruising around the house. Both are excited by the physical world and its many mysteries, both are intent on exploring, both push up against the limits of their own motor capabilities, trying to experience as much of the world as they can. Sandwiched between these two ages is the stage of Social Referencing, when infants were propelled by their newfound insights and concerns about the social world and their emerging capacities for integrating their concerns with those of other people. The 8- to 11-month-old infant was obsessed with his parents' whereabouts, the objects of their attention, and the bond between them. And he was obsessed with finding his parent when she disappeared. But the infant in the stages of Motor Initiative or Motor Practice is obsessed with the physical world and the wonderful opportunities it affords for exploring space and the objects within it. The stage of Motor Practice differs from previous stages as well. Most notably, there are now words to attach to objects, people, and simple properties and relationships. These words provide the child with surefire access to the attention and intentions of others, a way to call on them when in need, to share impressions and thoughts when desired, and generally to consolidate feelings of connection whenever he feels left out or insecure.

Sleep training at this stage gets a boost from the toddler's sense of autonomy, her interest in the nonsocial world, her relative independence and security, the robust and resilient nature of her emotions, and the sense of connection and social power she achieves through the beginnings of language. This is a relatively happy kid who can bounce back from emotional challenges, and one who is not so needy as to cling desperately to the image of a recently departed parent. However, sleep training at this age is also hampered by the 1-year-old's savvy. This kid has just emerged from a phase of relatively intense separation distress. Separations are no longer neutral. They are associated with feelings of loss, anxiety, sadness, and frustration. Although the peak intensity of separation reactions has passed by now, such reactions have not disappeared. Not at all. For the rest of her life, the child will never be entirely free of the potential for pain and anxiety that comes with being left alone and the sense of helplessness that goes with it.

The 12- to 16-month-old toddler may defy your efforts to change his bedtime routine. He may whine, or yell, or holler to get you back, aware of the power of his voice to bring you over that threshold once again. Stuffed animals will help. Music will help. Bedtime rituals, consisting of stories or songs, will help. This child, so autonomous an hour ago, needs to connect with you, needs to know that you are still within range. He needs to know that separation is not permanent, and that you're going to come back of your own accord. He needs to feel your love and your care, to know that he is the object of your attention and concern, and that he can call to you when it's time for reassurance. If you can balance these accommodations with the determination necessary to get him to go to sleep, most probably on his own, then sleep training at this age is likely to be successful.

Many of the pitfalls of sleep training at this age emerge from your child's spirit and her ingenuity. Her hands will find a way to make contact with every object on the dresser—that tube of cream, the box of tissues, the baby wipes, the pictures on the wall you thought were out of reach. Whether on her way to bed or once in bed, she will use every opportunity to play and explore rather than acquiesce to sleep. And she may be clever enough to capture you in her play. You may see this as bedtime, but for your toddler it's just another episode of playtime. And once you've said your last good night, you'll be amazed at the opportunities and reasons she finds to get you back. For example, she'll throw her stuffed animal to the floor and holler for you to bring it back to her—a seemingly legitimate reason to call on your sympathies. Whatever the obstacles you encounter, 12 to 16 months is a far easier time to initiate sleep training than either of the periods surrounding it. You just came from a stage of peak separation reactions combined with social referencing, and you're about to enter a stage when the toddler's whole emotional world is turned on its head, when defiance and autonomy compete with abject neediness and insecurity. In fact, if your child still isn't sleeping through the night, this may be your last chance for an efficient and fully satisfactory sleep-training experience. Life will get more complicated in a few more months, and even more complicated after that. The transition into the next stage is rapidly approaching, so get on with it!

> Many of the challenges of sleep training at this age involve your toddler's energetic spirit and intelligence.

Stage 7
Social Negotiation: 17 to 21 months

The period of 17 to 21 months, often considered the beginning of the Terrible Twos, is another tumultuous stage. As with the 8- to 11-month-old infant, sleep training at this age can result in more harm than good, and we strongly recommend waiting.

On the bright side, the period beginning at 17 to 18 months is a glorious phase of development. You will notice massive changes as your child moves beyond infancy into what can properly be called early childhood. As described in Chapter 2, language development begins to skyrocket as children learn to use two-part "sentences" that can describe exactly what they're thinking and what they want. They can also begin to understand social roles, conflicting goals, and other kinds of symbolic relationships, including simple rules and ideas such as cleanliness. These are huge cognitive changes, and indeed the 18-month transition is considered a major stage shift in many theories of cognitive development. But more than that, as described in Chapter 3, it is a period of emotional retooling. Children now begin to recognize themselves as beings in a truly *social* world made up of other people. They see themselves as individuals, with goals and wishes, and they see other people as individuals, also with goals and wishes. The realization that their wishes might just conflict with yours is an enormous challenge to what was previously a strong and superhero-like sense of self. Now they're not so sure whose wishes are going to prevail. As a result, conflicts grow in number and intensity, the word "No!" makes its debut, and toddlers try to establish a sense of security, balanced with a sense of independence, by commandeering their parents on some occasions, defying them on others, but always looking for signs of social approval, to reassure themselves that they are still members in good standing in the "club" of social connectedness. This is why we call this the period of Social Negotiation. Of course, such emotional changes can be difficult, but they are also touching and heartwarming. Your child is a real, independent little person now. With vulnerabilities and insecurities to be sure, but also with a new capacity for understanding and intimacy, and a kind of tenderness and love that we recognize as being very much like our own. Our babies are no longer tiny aliens: they are now complex social beings, with distinct personalities, needs, and ways of doing things.

What aspects of this period make it especially troublesome for sleep training? Separation is more painful now than it has been since the age of 8 to 11 months, because it is interpreted according to your baby's sense of *your* goals and agendas. If you are somewhere else, you could be intentionally ignoring him, perhaps because you have better things to do. Physical separation means psychological separation, and that is not a comforting option! In Figure 4 on page 154, you'll see the highest peak in separation distress at about 18 to 20 months, rising steadily from 16 months. Rather than being alone, the 18- to 20-month-old now wants to be with you . . . sometimes as much as possible. One mother had this to say about the emotional needs of this period.

DAWN'S STORY

Dramatic Cling

He's climbing all over me all the time, kicking and hitting and grabbing me while he nurses, screaming at me and demanding things he cannot ask for in words or signs, and hanging on to my legs as I try to walk . . . He's either giddy or distressed, in agony, about something.

And here is his latest: When I sit down on the toilet, he stands in front of me and grabs onto my knees and tries to climb into my pant legs with me. . . . He's so determined to be smashed up against me at every second. Eighteen months is busting my chops.

So what happens when you explain that it's time to go to sleep? You kiss your baby good night and tiptoe out of the room. You probably won't have to wait long before the first howling protest: "Nooooo! Come back! No sleep! Want kiss! Want hug! Want more! Get Daddy! Daddy come! Mommy come! Want Mommy, not Daddy. Want Daddy, not Mommy!" And on and on. This is precisely the social negotiation that you can expect at this age. Your child is using her collection of words to tell you what she wants, in as many ways as she can, knowing full well she's opposing your wishes. Her anxiety escalates as she realizes that you are becoming impatient and irritated. She therefore needs even more reassurance, making her increasingly determined not to be alone, as the struggle continues. Yet each time she tries another tactic, she feels like she's losing a little more of you. She is a little more in danger of being tossed out of the "club" of social closeness, or at the very least having her membership privileges revoked. And she *knows* it, but she can't stop, because to give in, to stop protesting, would mean accepting your absence and giving up her ability to enlist your care. If you disappear now, she's alone, really alone. And what's more, she is not very good at accepting defeat these days. Because not getting her way means a loss of her sense of power and effectiveness in the world in general and the social world in particular. And that feeling of helplessness is devastating.

The emotional changes that rapidly cascade from about 17 to 21 months are likely to make sleep training a dramatic, traumatic, and ultimately ineffective effort. And the reason for this is simple. During the period of Social Negotiation your baby is attempting to balance his needs for security, a sense of acceptance, and confidence in his parents' love on the one hand, with his need for independence and a sense of competence and accomplishment on the other. Your baby's attention is focused on conflicting goals and wishes. Frustration is met with tears, anger, and very often the first temper tantrums. For your child to give in and go to sleep would mean admitting defeat, which means relinquishing his sense of being important and effective. This is tantamount to having his newly established sense of power snatched away in one fell swoop. Indeed, sleep training at this age is bound to be hampered by two interlocking issues: your toddler's fear of separation and his determination to hold his own in conflict situations. Because of both issues, sleep training will be a hard-fought battle for the 17- to 21-month-old child. Here's how some parents have described their sleep standoffs at this age.

GERRY'S STORY

Pulling Out All the Stops

Monique is currently 18 months old and is still waking once a night. She's also become much harder to get down for both bedtime and naptime. I know that her verbal skills are growing exponentially—but, of course, she still can't tell me why she's waking or what's taking her so long to fall asleep!

We have never let her cry to get to sleep. She has rarely put herself to sleep. In most cases, there is singing or rocking or stories involved. And at bedtime, she still gets a bottle. But even these things don't seem to be enough to put her to sleep anymore. I've tried all the no-cry sleep solutions like the "pat, pick up, put down" method, but she's not getting it at all right now.

I'm just really tired of feeling like I've somehow failed her by not forcing her to fall asleep on her own or letting her cry it out. I already tried telling my mom that we will just have to disagree about Monique's sleep issues and not talk about it. But every time my mother brings it up, I feel superdefensive (especially when I get told, "I hope you don't nurse this next baby to sleep" and "I feel sorry for her; she obviously needs the sleep—she's overtired").

Our advice to Gerry? Wait it out. She is not a bad parent, no matter who tries to tell her so. She's made parenting decisions that suited her and her baby's needs, and they've worked so far. She should just hold out a little longer before trying to make any changes. By 22 months or so, Gerry can try the same gentle sleep-training methods she's been attempting, and Monique will probably respond quickly to the same efforts that seem so doomed right now.

As we can see from the next example, waiting it out can be difficult, but it helps to know that you're not alone.

MELANIE'S STORY

The Opposition Position

Eighteen months was probably the lowest point in my parenting career. . . . I actually thought my depression was coming back (the hormones of nursing made my depression disappear completely) because I just couldn't seem to grind through each day with a child who was smart and funny and loving, but fighting me at every turn.

He wouldn't nap. He went from sleeping all night to waking all night. He had a tantrum every 5 minutes, it seemed, mostly because he wanted to do everything himself and it just wasn't possible. He hardly ate. He whined. He never shared with the other kids, and he always tried to yank our cat's fur.

I was exhausted all the time and really doubting the decisions I'd made and my abilities as a mother. I think I could have dealt with the oppositional behavior (I knew in my head it was normal for that age), but not sleeping was killing me. Not only would our son not let my husband put him to sleep (starting almost exactly at 18 months), but he wanted to nurse every freaking time he woke up in the middle of the night. He went from sleeping from 8 p.m. to 6 a.m. to waking up three to five times a night for around a month. It made me want to run away.

And then, at around 20 months, it just suddenly went back to normal. He wanted Daddy to put him to sleep, and he slept through again. It certainly wasn't anything I did, because I was too fried to do anything but just try to make it through the day. The only consolation in all of it was that every single kid in our playgroup was doing the exact same thing, whether their parents had let them cry it out or not. Every one . . .

Stage 8
Social Stabilization: 22 to 27 months

Congratulations. You made it through the first onslaught of the Terrible Twos, the stage of Social Negotiation. If your baby still hasn't acquired healthy, stable sleep habits, then bedtimes have not been much fun for the last few months. And even if she has, they've probably become at least partially unraveled. The precocious, autonomous, demanding, yet insecure toddler of 18 to 20 months has been a handful, no doubt, and sleep habits were probably among the routines to take a serious hit. How many ways has your toddler acquired to verbalize her requirements for your presence at night? Has she learned yet to tell you that her blanket or soother has disappeared? What she didn't tell you is that she threw them on the floor to get you back. Our twins would chant, "Oh-oh soother!" or "Oh-oh blankie!" over and over, having just thrown these nighttime supplies as far as possible from their cribs until we reappeared in their room once again to pick them up. Eventually, we fought back with longer and longer periods of ignoring them, and they eventually gave it up. By 22 months or so, your child is more calm, more stable, and more secure than she was just recently. The massive cognitive changes ushered in by the stage of Roles, Goals, & Language have begun to consolidate. She has gotten used to being a social player in a social world. She understands what you require of her at mealtime and bedtime. Which means that she understands rules and can adapt to them if she has to. In short, she's ready for sleep training once again. But now it's important to introduce sleep training a little differently then you might have at younger ages. Now it can bear the stamp of a rule or obligation, because that's what 2-year-olds understand best.

By this age, sleep training is bound to be more complicated than it was during previous windows of opportunity. The cost-benefit analysis has got new issues stacked up on both sides. On the benefit side, you *really* need to get some sleep at night! And so does your kid. But more than that, the sorts of manipulations and ploys that 2-year-olds can muster can become a real drag for both of you. Your child is now motivated to exaggerate his needs for company in order to bring your goals into line with his. And his escalating complaints about how cold, or thirsty, or lonely he is become focal points in a dialogue that shouldn't even be taking place. Not after bedtime. What's more, these complaints may be as convincing to him as they are to you. As a result, he may use his mushrooming verbal abilities to talk himself into states of excessive neediness—not a particularly welcome turn of events for either of you. So the greatest benefit to sleep training now, rather than waiting even longer, is that your child needs clear limits in this emotional playing field, to avoid a gradual shift in his personality toward greater defiance, clinginess, whininess, or dependency in general. On the cost side, you're dealing with a child who is a lot smarter and more verbal than ever before. Driven by insecurity and anxiety about separations of any sort, he will put these skills to use as tools of manipulation, making him a formidable opponent in the great sleep wars. He is also a child who may have acquired serious negative associations to being left by himself, especially if he is temperamentally sensitive or anxious. He is smart enough to know that you have your own life to live, and your departure now signals that you really are finished playing for now—by your own volition. This social insight makes him more vulnerable to feelings of rejection than he was before 18 months. And hurt feelings are for real. So it's a tricky, more complex task at this age, but teaching your child healthy sleep habits can still be done, and done better now than in the next stage.

Sleep training the 2-year-old child will involve subtleties that were not at issue for younger children. Children this age (and older) see all social negotiations in terms of goals, roles, and the rules that apply to them. Families by now have begun to highlight rules, rehearse rule-appropriate behavior, and warn of consequences or other contingencies when rules are ignored or violated. It would be hard to implement sleep training in this period without bringing rules to mind, either explicitly or implicitly. A rule is, after all, a formula that connects an "if" to a "then." If x, then y. *If you eat your chicken, then you can have some blueberries. If you let me get your pyjamas on, then I'll read you a story. And if you stay in bed and quit hollering, then* . . . then what? And that's the problem. Even though going to bed and saying good night strongly resemble a rule, it isn't clear to the parent or the child what consequences will follow if the rule is opposed. There is no reward to offer subsequent to going to sleep. And we certainly wouldn't suggest implementing a punishment or consequence if the child remains obstinate. Bedtime is too emotionally sensitive, too laden with concerns and insecurities, to introduce any additional negative contingencies. But you're in luck. There is a natural contingency that you can take advantage of. Children in the stage of Social Stabilization are often eager to please their parents, and parental pleasure and approval might be enough of a reward to make going to sleep an attractive choice. Stuffed animals, stories, songs, and other bedtime rituals naturally sweeten the pot as well. These should be in plentiful supply.

Sleep training your 2-year-old child will inevitably involve highlighting rules and goals for her and the whole family.

Other subtleties involved in sleep training the 2- to 2½-year-old will no doubt become evident as you try your luck during this period. However, these will depend increasingly on your child's temperament, her coping skills, the particular constellation of your family, and other factors specific to each household. As far as temperament goes, the difficult child will be showing her true colors more in this stage than in previous windows. She may have much more intense emotional reactions to being left alone under any circumstances, including at night. She may be less likely to fall asleep, and less capable of yielding to any request, once her anxieties have been kindled; and the two of you may be accustomed to a higher pitch of argument and negotiation, setting the stage for lengthier confrontations at this most delicate moment in a day full of delicate moments. Whatever the case, however, the benefits will outweigh the costs for any child who still needs to acquire systematic sleep habits by this age.

Stage 9
Social Comparison: 28 months to 3 years

Typically, the period known as the Terrible Twos begins at 18 to 20 months, when children become more demanding and defiant, but the terribleness of toddlerhood often increases sharply at about the age of 2½ (28 to 30 months). In fact, many parents report that the Terrible Twos really start at this age. Children become more clever. They can imagine more than one social relationship at the same time, such as the relationship between achieving versus failing a goal and the relationship between following versus breaking a rule. This means that they can weigh the impact of their rule-breaking behavior on your goals, your wishes, and ultimately your feelings. We discussed this in some depth last chapter, but there are other examples of Social Comparison, including the capacity to play one parent off against another: *If I ask my dad for a cookie, I'm likely to get one. If I ask my mom, I'm not likely to get one. So I'll wait till Dad comes back.* Children become more manipulative, perhaps more sly. They test the limits in new and more subtle ways, because they understand social rules very well by now, and they know that breaking rules is one sure way to bug you. We could say that the typical 2½-year-old is a terribly cute little criminal concerned mostly with getting caught, rather than with the act itself. But despite their rambunctiousness, these children have one primary weakness: jealousy. This is the age at which it begins. As we discussed in Chapter 3, the ability to compare two social relationships allows children to feel that their relationship with you is compromised by your relationship with someone else. This someone else could be another sibling, or it could be your husband. Whatever the case, jealousy is among the most painful of emotions, and the capacity to feel it is like an Achilles heel to a 2½-year-old.

It is a little more difficult to talk about this period of development in definitive terms, because individual differences become more pronounced by this age, and what we might call a typical pattern of development becomes more blurred. Jealousy is a perfect example. Some children are highly sensitive to jealous feelings, and their sensitivity may result from temperament, from the fact of having a younger sibling to compete with, or from a combination of the two. Similarly, the degree of defiance and testing of limits varies hugely from child to child. At 2½ to 3 years of age, some children are more concerned with "being good" than anything else. They love the praise, warmth, and other rewards that come from winning their parents' approval. Others are little devils who seem capable of finding the gray areas in any household rules and exploiting them to unpredictable extremes. Some children remain in steady control of their emotions, but many can be explosive, and temper tantrums at this age can be long, drawn-out affairs that tax the strength of even veteran parents.

Because of this variability, our advice about sleep training has to be more tailored at this age. We suggest you give sleep training a pass for several months if your child is prone to jealousy, if he is on the defiant end of the spectrum, or if he tends to wage battles whenever rules and regulations are not carved in stone. These emotional hot spots will become more muted soon, often by the age of 3 years. Instead, work on upgrading your discipline practices. Once your child is cooperating more than fighting you, everything will get easier—including sleep training. Also, take advantage of familiar routines and nightly rituals, including reading and telling stories, as these often maximize comfort and closeness for children who are emotionally volatile. But if your child has an easier disposition, if he already seems comfortable and relaxed about his role in the family, it might not be necessary to wait any longer. You have to make the call.

Let's imagine a child who is prone to jealousy. What is likely to go wrong if you try to alter her sleep habits at this age? She is used to falling asleep in your bed and then being carried back to her room when she's sound asleep. She's in the habit of strolling back to your bed a couple of times a night, and each time you wonder whether it's worth it to carry her back to her bed. Now let's imagine you have a new baby. Or maybe you just want a little more romance in your life. So you begin to insist that your daughter fall asleep in her own bed. You read her a quick story and say good night. A child who is struggling with feelings of jealousy will fight you tooth and nail. If there's a little baby in your bed these days, that means you prefer the baby to her, and there's no way she's going to stand for that! But even the sounds of you and your spouse talking together quietly, or giggling, or other signs of mutual enjoyment will be enough to catapult her out of her bed and back into yours. She does not want to be left out, she wants to be important, and special, and even powerful, and she needs to show you that she is just as lovable as she ever was. Fighting these jealous reactions through bribery, harsh words, or escalating punishments is going to sap your emotional strength just as it raises the stakes for your daughter and erodes her sense of well-being. It is far wiser to let her persist in her bad habits, at least for now, until she feels big enough, loved enough, and secure enough to fall asleep on her own, roughly by the age of 3 years.

> The capacity to feel intense jealousy
> can make 28 to 36 months a difficult
> period for sleep training.

Stage 10
Family Membership: 3 to 3½ years

This is the last window of opportunity to initiate or repair sleep habits for your child. By this time, most families will have already implemented sleep training of one kind or another, unless graced with one of those rare children who start sleeping through the night on their own. So this probably isn't your first shot at it. What's more likely is that you tried a sleep-training method that just didn't work for you, or you tried sleep training at an age when the deck was stacked against you. One way or another, sleep training didn't work in the past, or it worked for a while and then fell apart. And now you're looking at a kid who isn't a baby anymore—not by any stretch of the imagination—and who really shouldn't *need* your ministrations for very long in order to get to sleep and stay asleep for the night. It may also be the case that you're expecting another child, or a sibling has already been introduced to the family mix, a baby who needs pretty much all the resources you can muster, and you just don't have it in you to continue to negotiate sleep issues with your 3-year-old. And this child is a master negotiator by now. His understanding of family roles and his place within them has become highly sophisticated. He knows how to follow or break rules in order to win your approval or press your buttons. He has become well versed in the arts of familial diplomacy. And his recent peak in feelings of jealousy have left him more guarded than you might have wished. A little more determined to carve out some safe territory for himself. And this territory might include his hold on your emotions when it comes to dicey issues like separation and loss.

Nevertheless, the stage of Family Membership represents your last chance to sleep train before things become even more difficult: when false-belief understanding makes its appearance in the stage of Self-consciousness. Last chapter, we explained in detail why you should probably avoid sleep training once your child begins to see you as having your own private thoughts and opinions, because that insight opens the door to a new set of concerns—concerns that you might see her in a negative light. The resulting feelings of self-consciousness and shame make any social disengagement potentially fraught with new insecurities, especially when it involves leaving your child to ruminate by herself in the dark. So it is very important to set in place a viable set of bedtime habits before the stage of Self-consciousness begins. On the positive side, there are ways in which the current stage, though definitely late in the game, provides unique advantages that can ease the sleep-training process. As the name *Family Membership* implies, your child now sees herself, first of all, as a member of the family: one who wants to remain in good standing and who has the necessary skills to manipulate your thoughts, your moods, and your feelings in order to do so, essentially by being a "good" little girl and playing by the rules. So there is a distinct motivation built in at this age to get along, even before the withering concerns of self-consciousness raise the stakes a few months from now. And the will to get along, to be "good," and to make parents happy can be an important ally in the struggle for a lasting good night.

> Around 3 to 3½ years of age is the last chance to sleep train before the very dicey period of self-consciousness comes online.

Your child is highly aware of role relationships within the family, and this preoccupation manifests itself in a surge of family themes in his pretend play. You may notice that your 3-year-old, who has been engaged in "socio-dramatic" play for at least half a year to a year, now brings to this play a new level of richness. His animals or "men" or dolls have personalities that express their family roles: there is the daddy dinosaur and the mommy dinosaur, and their job is to feed all the little baby dinosaurs. The dolls are talking to each other about what to serve for dinner. They consult with each other about the little dinosaur's bad behavior. Should he be sent to his room for a time-out? The favorite animals—those elite few who sleep cheek-to-cheek with your child at night—are especially invested with role-specific personalities, and usually several at a time. Most interesting, these personalities can be largely incompatible, but each takes the stage for a time. So animals and dolls can take on different roles depending on what the situation demands. Now when the situation is bedtime, stuffed animals and their ilk become highly valuable sources of comfort for the 3-year-old child. Marc remembers Zoe's behavior at this age and the many intimate, intense, and sometimes contentious debates with Doggie, her favorite stuffed animal, once the lights had been turned out. But most of all, Doggie was a source of affection and connection for Zoe. Doggie's nose had become a highly polished nub by Zoe's middle childhood because of the nightly rubbing it received. In fact, Doggie invariably went to sleep nuzzled against Zoe's chin, and that made it a lot easier for her father to say good night and mean it.

These features of 3-year-old social intelligence will be of some help to you in sleep training your child. But of course, once again, differences in temperament and family constellation make it impossible to provide an all-purpose cookbook, or an almanac for predicting success versus failure. So we end this section with a reminder that the stage of Family Membership is something of a last chance. Sleep habits can be taught and retaught at any age. There is little doubt that you'll be engaged in negotiations around bedtime when your child is 13, 14, or 15 years old. But once false-belief understanding, with its accompanying dynamics of self-consciousness and shame, enter the mix by the age of 4 years, the psychological issues that impact on sleep training become considerably more complicated and potentially distressing, from early childhood on up through the age span. Take advantage of this last window of opportunity and bite the bullet before things get more difficult.

Stage 11
Self-consciousness: 3½ to 4 years

This is the final period we'll discuss as being potentially difficult for sleep training. It should be clear by now that if you still aren't getting your child to fall asleep and stay asleep without intervention, you're running late! There are plenty of windows of opportunity for sleep training in the first 3½ years, and we hope you've taken advantage of at least one of them. But if you haven't, or if for some reason your child's sleep habits have taken a turn for the worse, then the period of 3½ to 4 years may not be the ideal time to start or to restart your engines. Again, there are major individual differences by this age that make it difficult to provide a one-size-fits-all prescription. But there is one developmental issue that is likely to have considerable impact for any child. It's a big one, and its ramifications extend into many facets of your child's emotional life.

The issue, of course, is false-belief understanding, which we cover in some detail in Chapters 2 and 3. During this age range most normal children first develop the concept that other people have minds of their own. This acquisition of a theory of mind means that children now view other people, including their parents, as having sets of beliefs. Other people don't necessarily see things the way they do, and they now understand that the way people interpret things depends on their sources of information. Recall Bert and Ernie and the placement of the chocolates in the second of two hiding places. That scenario showed us that by the age of 3½ to 4 years, children understand that other people, and especially parents, can think things that aren't true. In other words, they can have false beliefs. We explain in Chapter

3 that the emotional consequences of false-belief understanding encompass heightened shame reactions. Examples include children who, after months of friendly greetings when their parents come upon them unexpectedly, suddenly shout, "Don't look at me!" or "Don't listen to my song!" or "Close the door!" so that they won't have to be exposed to their parents' scrutiny—even though this scrutiny is largely imagined. Children at this age, and especially those who are more sensitive temperamentally, just don't want to be seen when they feel vulnerable, and they feel especially vulnerable when they imagine that their thoughts or feelings might be viewed as "bad" or inappropriate. They also begin to show other insecurities at this age, including anxieties about others being angry at them and less explicit fears and concerns. Because shame and anxiety are such powerful emotions, any major change in your bedtime policies—especially one that leaves your child alone to ruminate for a while—can potentially produce a cascade of unwanted effects. We therefore suggest that parents carefully gauge their child's temperamental sensitivity or vulnerability if they are considering sleep training at this age.

Feelings of shame can be debilitating for some children around 3½ years old; sleep training should be avoided for these sensitive kids.

Sleep training after the age of 3 is less likely to involve crying spells or other extreme emotional displays. But it may evoke more subtle emotional reactions that are just as disturbing. What is your child feeling while lying in bed, waiting for sleep to come? Is he feeling ashamed of something he felt or did? Does he wonder if being left alone reflects your disapproval, your wish to be rid of him? He now has the capacity to imagine that you are thinking just about anything, and a young child's imagination can go to extremes that you and I would find remarkable and frightening. Children have plenty of time to mull over what their parents might be thinking about them while they are lying in bed alone. And if those thoughts include images of rejection, disapproval, or even abandonment, then they may lead to habitual worries that will eventually crystallize into long-lasting insecurities. Remember that these insecurities can emerge without much fanfare but settle in over time and endure for years. Yet, shame and insecurity are never invisible. Your child will let you know by word or deed if he feels rejected, as long as you are tuned in enough to notice. If he asks why he can't sleep with you anymore, it would be important to reassure him that it has nothing to do with his qualities. It's not about his being bad, or mean, or babyish, or selfish. (Of course, don't raise these issues by name if he doesn't!) Rather, let him know that it's about being a big boy and having a chance to read his own books, or turn off the lights by himself, or whatever may seem to enhance his self-esteem. This kind of reassurance can go a long way during this period of emotional uncertainty.

The volatile period when children acquire false-belief understanding may be short-lived (see Chapter 3). We view this period as a transitional phase, during which new cognitive interpretations give rise to novel and often troubling emotional constellations that have not yet been countered by coping responses. These coping responses will soon develop and will pave the way for social perceptions that are both insightful and flexible. And when these coping responses have stabilized, the insecurities of this period will recede into the background once again. Once you notice these improvements, perhaps after a few months, you may decide to be more ambitious in your attempts to adjust behavioral habits, including sleep training. In fact, especially if your child is temperamentally "easy," coming up on the age of 4 years can be a good time to take advantage of his newfound concern for the opinions of others. Now you can allow him to reflect on the fact that you do disapprove of some behaviors more than others. That will give you an important advantage in the ongoing struggle to raise a child who is well-behaved and pleasant to be with, as well as confident and secure.

This completes our advice for parents on the basis of contemporary developmental theory, research on parent–child interactions, and the common sense we've acquired from being connected to these literatures. As mentioned at the end of Chapter 3, we are aware that our predictions of age-specific issues for sleep training may be problematic for some families. There is enormous individual variation in children's mental, emotional, and behavioral tendencies. Every child's habits will vary to at least some degree from the idealized version we describe at each stage. Only your insights as a parent and the deep understanding you've acquired about your own child's personality and cognitive and emotional development will provide the appropriate modifications to the "average" timetable we've provided.

5

The Pros and Cons of Popular Sleep-Training Methods

WE BELIEVE THAT THE *AGE AND STAGE* YOU CHOOSE to teach your young child to sleep is just as important as the method you use. Perhaps more important. But if you haven't already found this out, deciding what method to use turns out to be a critical decision as well—a very personal and powerfully emotional decision at that. How to teach your child to sleep better (whatever that definition is for you), assuming you believe that's a lesson that ought to be learned, is among the most hotly debated issues among new parents. And of course there are strongly held beliefs and philosophies about the diverse sleep-training experts.

Ideally, there should be strong empirical support for at least one of the many methods out there but, in fact, this area of research is rather dismal. We'll save you the details and simply point you to one interesting recent review of the most popular sleep-training methods, conducted by the American Academy of Sleep Medicine (published in 2006 in the journal *Sleep*). The review concluded that no sleep-training method is superior to any other in terms of effectiveness. That's right: the surprising conclusion was that there's no one best way to do it. Instead, the key is consistency. Whatever method you choose, use it consistently. We would add, of course, apply your preferred method during the right developmental window.

No systematic studies have been conducted to identify the best sleep-training method.

The five most popular sleep-training techniques can be categorized roughly on a continuum from least intervention (leaving the child alone in her room) to most intervention (holding the child and providing maximum comfort). Another way to characterize this continuum is to say that it ranges from methods that advocate letting children cry themselves to sleep to methods that try to avoid any crying at all.

Despite raging debates, most authors of sleep-training books share the goal of providing children with warm, relaxing rituals that will make it easy for them to *want* to go to sleep. Most think bedtime should be a time for parents and children to feel close and secure with one another. Almost all the sleep-training manuals out there advise parents first and foremost to set up regular bedtime rituals that will reliably signal the baby or toddler that it is time to go to sleep. Most of these rituals include some variation of feeding the baby (either nursing or bottle-feeding), giving a warm, soothing bath, perhaps reading a bedtime story or two, singing or playing lullabies, and then, finally, putting the child down in his crib (or family bed).

The methods begin to diverge at this point. We start with the least-intervention end of the continuum and follow the methods through to the other end.

Cry-It-Out

Cry-it-out methods, also referred to as "extinction," are strategies that advocate putting your child to bed by herself and letting her fall asleep on her own. Most babies don't do this right away, so this method encourages parents to let the baby cry until she does eventually fall asleep, whether that takes 10 minutes or 3 hours. The full-out cry-it-out strategy requires parents to make sure the baby is fed, warm, and dry, and then to leave the baby alone and refrain from checking in on her while this training is in process.

The philosophy behind this methodology (and the more gradual extinction method that follows) is that babies need to learn how to soothe themselves to sleep, and that if we don't allow them that opportunity, they will never learn the skill. If a mother nurses, rocks, bounces, or sings her baby to sleep, then the baby learns to fall asleep using those props. When the baby wakes up partially or completely in the middle of the night, as all of us do (not just infants), then he no longer has those props to help him fall back to sleep and he wakes up the rest of the way, crying. If, on the other hand, the baby learns to put himself to sleep by sucking his thumb, humming to himself, attending to a mobile, and so on, then when he wakes up in the middle of the night he'll be able to self-soothe and get himself back to sleep without assistance from mother.

A small detour here: There is nothing wrong with rocking or nursing or soothing your baby to sleep. As many parents will attest (including ourselves), the bedtime rituals for putting young babies to sleep can be the most treasured, most magical times in the early months of child-rearing. There really is nothing like looking down at your peacefully sleeping infant, feeling her breath against your arm, her warmth seep into your body. We have both had the pleasure of falling asleep ourselves with one of our boys tucked into our necks. It's heaven. We are in no way suggesting that these rituals aren't precious or worth keeping in those early months or even years. However, many parents eventually can't take the sleep deprivation that usually goes along with extended periods of this arrangement. As a result, they resort to some sort of sleep-training procedure. So, enjoy the rocking, singing, and nursing that helps get your baby to sleep. Enjoy it for as long as it feels right for you and your family. And then, if or when it's not working for you anymore, either because you're blind with fatigue or because your child has decided she'd rather play trampoline on mommy than be rocked back to sleep, it's time for a change. Babies and toddlers are malleable little beings and they can learn and unlearn habits with reasonable ease, especially if we target these lessons for the right developmental window.

Don't worry that you've created "bad" sleep habits: babies can learn new strategies with remarkable ease, as long as we teach them during the right developmental window.

Contrary to misinterpretations and media hype, Richard Ferber is not an advocate of the cry-it-out approach, although his name is most commonly associated with it. (We'll talk more about Ferber in the next section.) Jodi Mindell, in her book *Sleeping Through the Night: How Infants, Toddlers, and Their Parents Can Get a Good Night's Sleep,* suggests cry-it-out as one of many strategies that might be effective for some families. Her book is chockful of research on children's sleep patterns, and she comes with strong credentials. Marc Weissbluth's *Healthy Sleep Habits, Happy Child* also suggests this as one of two methods for getting your child to sleep through the night or nap sufficiently during the day. Weissbluth's advice is more extensive, however, and only mentions extinction as one possible, often last-ditch, effort at sleep training.

In terms of the actual "how to" of this method, there really is no technique as such. You just put your baby down in his crib or bassinette when he is sleepy but still awake. After saying your good nights, you close the door and leave him alone. Most babies at this point will start crying, and the duration of that crying will depend on how terrible the experience feels for him (and you). We suggest that the duration of crying is highly dependent on developmental timing, so we advise a careful consideration of optimal windows if you're going the cry-it-out route.

Many parents who advocate this method do so because it can be very efficient and effective for some children and it actually ends up saving a lot more tears than it produces, again for *some* children. Countless parents report letting their child cry it out as a last resort, after many failed efforts with different, more gentle approaches. Most parents who have succeeded with this method report that if they tried to go back into the room to soothe their baby before she fell asleep, the crying would only escalate.

The Clean Break

It felt like I was teasing the baby. She would be crying for 10 minutes, at which point I'd walk back into the room to pat her, reassure her with "I love you," shush to her softly, and then I'd leave. She'd calm down a little when I was in the room, but as soon as she'd see me walking out again, she'd wail bloody murder. Each time I came back in after that, she'd cry even harder than when I was gone. Finally I just felt like I was torturing her (and me!) each time I went in, so I stopped. I just decided I wouldn't go back in at all after I put her down. That first night, she cried off and on for 90 minutes. The next night she cried again for about 90 minutes. Those were terrible, terrible nights. I felt like a failure, like I was being cruel to my baby. But the only thing that helped me keep going was that it was actually *less* crying in total than the nights when I'd go in and out a million times. The third night, I still didn't go back in, but this time she fell asleep after 50 minutes. Finally, on the fourth night, I put my baby down and she didn't even whimper. After about 5 minutes, I went in to check on her, and she was fast asleep. She's been sleeping through the night ever since.

Like Jessica, many parents who let their baby cry it out report that it was a heart-wrenching process. Sometimes infants cry for up to 3 hours before falling asleep the first night. But then, gradually, there is a decline in the duration of crying, and usually by the end of a week or so, most babies will have stopped crying altogether, or cry very little, before falling asleep on their own. Oftentimes this spells the end of night wakings entirely. Advocates of this approach insist that their children were crying far more hours when they were being soothed to sleep by their parents, or when they were waking up every hour over the course of the night. Also, parents successful with this method report that their children are far happier, more energetic, less lethargic, and less hyperactive. In other words, for some families who can tolerate crying for some period of time without intervention, this method may be the quickest route to getting the whole family some much-needed rest.

Parents and experts who argue against this approach say that letting a child cry herself to sleep is not actually teaching a skill at all. Instead, the child is learning that parents can become inexplicably inaccessible during some of the most scary times of their lives. Critics of cry-it-out suggest that children who are left to sob themselves to sleep will eventually grow up insecure and less "attached" to their parents. Although we sympathize with the feelings underlying these arguments, there is no empirical support for the claim that children are "damaged" by cry-it-out methods. In fact, there are several studies in reputable psychological and pediatric journals that suggest no long-term harmful effects on children whose parents let them cry for periods of time while sleep training.

In summary, there are both pros and cons to the cry-it-out approach. Ultimately, it is up to you to weigh these sides for your family's needs. The only suggestion we make in terms of this method (and we advise the same for any method that advocates leaving a child alone to self-soothe) is that you should not let a baby cry himself to sleep for any more than 1 or 2 minutes before around 2½ months. As we describe in earlier chapters, babies are still working on getting their biological states and rhythms synchronized, and they aren't able to regulate their own arousal levels. So, most infants younger than 3 months can't bring themselves back down on their own once they've started to cry uncontrollably. They also still need to be fed during the night, and their cries of hunger may be misread as cries of protest. Finally, the mother is just beginning to read the myriad signals the new baby is sending her, both during the day and at night, as her own patterns and rhythms become synchronized with those of her baby. Letting your infant cry without responding at such an early age may truncate that critical phase of bonding and synchronization. Although we understand why some parents choose this method, and it may indeed be the best one for you, we suggest waiting until the baby is at least 3 months of age—and ideally until about 6 months old.

Gradual Extinction, or "Ferberizing"

Perhaps the most widely known sleep-training method is Richard Ferber's progressive approach to teaching children to sleep on their own. "Ferberizing" is a deceptively simple method that uses basic behavioral principles to help babies gradually take on the task of putting themselves to sleep. Contrary to misrepresentations of the Ferber method, it was developed as an *alternative* to the full-blown cry-it-out technique. Instead of allowing the baby to cry for however long it takes until she falls asleep on her own, Ferber advocates a gradual weaning of parental support.

The rationale for Ferber's approach is the same one we've outlined for full-blown cry-it-out methods. Ferber and other sleep experts believe that from around the age of 6 months, most children no longer need to wake up in the middle of the night to be fed—they can get all the nutrition they need during the day. So, at around this early age, your child can be taught to put himself to sleep.

The goal of Ferber's method is to teach the child to fall asleep on her own without parental props and support.

Six months happens to be an ideal developmental window for sleep training, as discussed in Chapter 3 and especially Chapter 4. If you're like many parents, up to this age, you've been rocking, gliding, nursing, singing, or bouncing your infant for extended periods of time before she falls deeply asleep in your arms. Then you ever so gently lay her in her crib, taking great care to move your hands slowly from under her head and stealthily back out of the nursery. As you gingerly inch the door closed . . . your baby suddenly jolts from her slumber with a wail that could wake the dead. And then she is inconsolable and unable to go back to sleep. So you start the process of rocking, gliding, nursing, singing, or bouncing all over again. The same thing happens 2 hours later when she wakes in the night, and an hour after that, and an hour after that. The problem, says Ferber, is that your baby has built up very particular sleep associations that include her mother's presence, lots of cuddling, and lots of movement. All of these conditions are unavailable to the baby when she wakes or partially wakes in the middle of the night. Of course she calls out for you so that you can yet again help her fall asleep with the props she's grown used to. In essence, those children who fall asleep in one context (for example, on Mama's breast) and wake up in another (for example, alone in a crib) will start crying because they're confused and scared and can't bring back the context that put them to sleep in the first place. Ferber suggests parents imagine what it would feel like to go to sleep in your bed and wake up in the garage: disturbing to say the least. So the goal of Ferber's method is for the parent gradually to transfer an extensive arsenal of sleep supports to the child herself.

"Ferberizing" is a simple method that involves several straightforward steps:

1. Put your child in his crib sleepy, but still awake.
2. Say your comforting good nights and then leave the room.
3. At this point the child will usually begin to cry if he is not used to being left alone to soothe himself.
4. After an initial, short, predetermined duration (for

example, after 3 minutes), return to the child. Pat him, say soothing words, stroke his back or belly, but do not pick him up. Stay in the room for only 1 to 2 minutes and then promptly leave again.

5. Increase the period of time that you leave the child to fuss or cry before you return to soothe him, always without picking him up (for example, return after 5 minutes, then 7 minutes, then 10 minutes, and so on). Each time, leave the room after 1 to 2 minutes of soothing.

6. Incrementally increase the duration of time you stay out of the room while your child attempts to put himself to sleep (or, as is often the case for the first day or two, cries his little head off). Eventually, he will fall asleep on his own.

After about a week or two, Ferber says, most babies will learn to soothe themselves both at bedtime and when they awaken during the night.

The most important advice about Ferberizing is to follow the method *consistently*. This message is relevant for all sleep-training methods, but perhaps most important for this one. The reason goes back to basic principles of behavioral psychology. Over and over, psychologists have discovered that "intermittent" reinforcement—reinforcing a behavior by rewarding it unpredictably—is the *best* way to create a stable behavioral habit. Unpredictable reinforcement creates even stronger habits than consistently reinforcing a behavior. That's because the uncertainty of whether the reward will be coming this time or next keeps the goal of attaining that reward in the forefront of the baby's mind (or the mind of any animal, for that matter). If you sometimes return immediately (when the baby's cries become too much for you to bear) and you stay out of the room for long stretches at other times, there is no predictability to the rewards your baby is receiving. Without any predictable schedule of soothing, the baby may continue to cry longer until she gets you back. Alternatively, if you follow Ferber's schedule and return to the baby to soothe and cuddle, but at ever-increasing durations, the child learns that escalating her crying will not bring you back any sooner. If this method is followed consistently, most babies learn the game of increasing durations quickly, over just a few days. They learn that they will have to use their own resources to go to sleep because, although Mommy is out there and has not disappeared, she will not come back just because her baby is crying.

There are several reasons to recommend this gradual extinction method, or "Ferberizing." Most important, unlike with full-blown cry-it-out methods, with this one parents can feel like they are reassuring their child as the child is learning the ropes of falling asleep on his own. Because parents can start by checking on their child even after 1 or 2 minutes, increasing the duration from there, this approach often seems much more gentle than leaving the baby alone to cry himself to sleep. In fact, this method is probably meant to reassure the parent as much, or more than, the child during this difficult training process. Second, Ferber has a reasonable amount of empirical evidence to back up his claims that the method works, and works for *most* children, if implemented correctly. Third, if you read the second edition of Ferber's book, *How to Solve Your Child's*

Sleep Problems, the author provides extensive information on how first to diagnose the barriers to getting your child to sleep on his own (for example, teething or illness). As a result, you can tailor the gradual extinction method to match the needs of your child.

OLYMPIA'S STORY

Rinse and Repeat

"Ferberizing" saved our lives . . . and definitely our sanity. I had been nursing the bub to sleep for the first 6 months of his life. It was often a beautiful, peaceful experience the first time he'd go down for the night. But progressively, I started to resent him more and more, as he'd wake up throughout the night. I'd feel guilty about how angry I was at him, because it was always my dream to be able to cuddle with my baby, breast-feed him, and then watch him sleep peacefully in my arms. That dream gradually turned into a nightmare when I was getting 2 to 3 hours of sleep per night. We'd nurse and rock and snuggle, and he'd be fast asleep, and the millisecond I'd put him down in the crib, up he'd spring. Rinse, repeat, over and over and over through the night. Teaching some self-soothing skills became critical for us. It took exactly two nights, a total of 20 minutes of crying and three check-ins to comfort him and let him know that we hadn't disappeared off the planet. Just like that, it worked, and now he wakes up and cries for me only when there's really something wrong (and then, of course, I go to him immediately). There is no doubt in our minds that we made the right choice.

Of course, there are also reasons to be cautious about this sleep-training technique. First, it *does* require the parent to ignore (or at least refrain from responding to) her baby's cries. Although there's a chance to return to the child at regular intervals, hearing her distressed cries just seems unbearable to some parents. As a result, many find it difficult to keep to a predictable schedule that maintains an ever-increasing duration between visits to the baby's crib. Without this consistency, the method is likely to fail, and many parents will then give up, sometimes after just a day or two. Second, like all methods, it doesn't work for all babies. For some, the repeated visits from the parent serve to increase frustration and result in escalations in crying. These may lead to uncontrollable sobbing and even throwing up. For those perhaps more sensitive children, even implementing this method consistently won't decrease the duration of crying before sleep. Third, this method may work best for children younger than about 16 months. As reviewed in detail earlier, after children hit the 18-month stage transition, they "wake up" socially, separation distress peaks again, their language skills become sophisticated, and they are emotionally much more complex than before. As a result, they may not "fall for" the Ferberizing method in the same way that younger children do. Given their increased working memory capacity, older children may realize that, no matter what, Mom will return eventually, especially if they stay awake and cry. Thus the usefulness of this method may be limited to the first year and a half of life.

Sleep Routines and Scheduling

Another approach to sleep training involves creating good sleep habits from a very young age. There is no precise name for this method, but it focuses on putting babies on sleeping and feeding schedules that promote children's capacity to sleep through the night and nap regularly. Perhaps the best-known manual for this approach is Weissbluth's *Healthy Sleep Habits, Happy Child.* But in truth, most grandmothers with lots of experience in child-rearing have given the same advice for decades, probably centuries.

The rationale is that babies and toddlers have natural, neurologically based sleep rhythms that should be respected. It is the parents' job to structure the child's day and night such that sleep is optimized. The goal is to get babies and toddlers to sleep for age-appropriate durations throughout the day and night by watching the baby's cues and following a handful of tips. Some may be counterintuitive, but they are all "tried and true" techniques.

- Sleep begets sleep. The more a child naps during the day, the more likely he will sleep longer and wake less frequently during the night.
- If a child is waking up frequently during the night or waking up far too early, put the child to sleep *earlier* at night (rather than the more intuitive later bedtime).
- Do not allow babies younger than 4 months or so to stay awake for more than 1 to 2 hours at a time during the day.
- Watch for telltale signs of fatigue and put your baby down for a nap or for bedtime as soon as you see these signs (even

if they occur only 1 hour after the baby has woken up). The sleepy signs include the baby rubbing his eyes, yawning, batting his ears, whining or fussing, and so on.

- Use the same bedtime routine every night (often including bath, bottle, breast-feeding, stories, rocking, and so on).

Another tip comes from a number of online sources, the origins of which are difficult to pinpoint. We came upon it on the parenting blog AskMoxie.com. It's called the 2–3–4 Rule and an astonishing number of babies between the ages of about 6 and 18 months end up conforming to this rule. Keeping it in mind was enormously helpful for scheduling our boys' naps. The idea is that 2 hours after the baby wakes up in the morning, you put him down for his first nap (whether you see signs of fatigue or not). Then, 3 hours after he wakes from that first nap, you put him down for his second nap. Then, 4 hours after he wakes from that second nap, you put him down for the night. So, for babies who sleep at night from approximately 7 p.m. until 7 a.m. (a recommended period, although often an unattainable goal), the sleep and wake periods fall out roughly as follows:

7 a.m.   wake for the day

9 a.m.   first nap

10 a.m.   wake from first nap

1 p.m.   second nap

3 p.m.   wake from second nap

7 p.m.   bedtime

Generally, after the child has reached 12 to 18 months, he drops the first morning nap. The afternoon nap can then get a little longer and start a little earlier.

Gentle or No-Cry Methods

One set of methods is often referred to as "no-cry" solutions, from Elizabeth Pantley's popular book by the same name, *The No-Cry Sleep Solution: Gentle Ways to Help Your Baby Sleep Through the Night.* The methods under the rubric of "attachment parenting" would also be classified as gentle methods, including manuals such as William Sears's *Nighttime Parenting* and James J. McKenna's *Sleeping with Your Baby: A Parent's Guide to Co-Sleeping.* What these approaches have in common is a commitment to minimizing or altogether eliminating any distress at all in your baby when she is falling asleep for naps or bedtime. The Sears and McKenna approaches focus particularly on encouraging co-sleeping practices. Sears is well recognized for encouraging parents to accept the natural, often difficult sleep patterns that many babies and toddlers fall into in the first 2 years of life. He stresses that parents can't "force" their children to sleep longer stretches. He and other attachment-parenting gurus suggest that sleep training itself is not a healthy, productive way to promote healthy sleep habits. Instead, parents should learn to structure their lives such that their own sleep is maximized, but be realistic and understand that sleep deprivation in the first few years of parenting is simply a part of the experience.

Proponents of gentle or no-cry methods of putting your child to sleep argue that for centuries and across many cultures mothers have kept their babies and toddlers as close as possible to their bodies. Co-sleeping and "wearing" your baby are examples of critical practices that promote a healthy bond between the mother and child, a bond necessary for the child's optimal development. These authors go on to argue that mothers who systematically ignore their babies' cries during the night foster deep anxieties and insecurities that will leave the child with emotional scars for life. Here are some of the most common sleep strategies often touted as "attachment" oriented:

- Sleep with your child in the same bed (co-sleep).
- "Wear" your baby (in a sling or other type of baby carrier) as much as possible throughout the day and at night if necessary.
- Nurse on demand, and particularly before naptimes and bedtimes, to help the baby fall asleep peacefully.
- Fathers can bounce, rock, or cuddle the baby into a deep sleep.
- If you leave the baby alone in a crib or bassinet, leave behind an article of clothing or cloth that carries the mother's scent.
- Respond as quickly as possible to your child's cries at bedtime and throughout the night (in other words, try not to let your child cry for any length of time before falling asleep or upon waking during the night).

Pantley's "no-cry" solutions are also geared toward minimizing children's distress, and her approach is meant as an alternative to the cry-it-out methods. In addition to her other commonsense suggestions, including creating a relaxing atmosphere (e.g., dim lighting), providing a bedtime ritual, and so on, Pantley offers a number of tips. Hers is not a sleep-training method as such, but a set of helpful soothing strategies aimed at transitioning children's bedtime and napping habits gradually. For example, if a parent wants to stop nursing her baby to sleep, Pantley suggests substituting the nursing with gentle rocking, then the rocking with patting in the crib, and then finally moving toward putting the child down on her own to see if she'll self-soothe. Other examples include a form of "gradual extinction" but at a much slower pace than in Ferber's approach. To get a child to fall asleep on her own, in her crib, on the first night a parent might sit close to the child with a hand on her child's belly and stay that way until she falls asleep. The next night, the parent may move the chair back a yard or so and not touch the child. The next night, the parent may inch the chair back even farther, and so on, until eventually she is outside the child's room and the child can fall asleep on her own.

> No-cry techniques were developed by authors who saw a need for alternatives to cry-it-out solutions.

Another popular "gentle" sleep-training method comes from Tracy Hogg's *The Baby Whisperer* approach. This technique, often referred to as the "shush/pat" method, is meant to be a soothing, gradual way to help your child learn to fall asleep on his own. The basic steps are as follows:

1. Make the room in which the baby will be sleeping as dark as possible.
2. Swaddle the baby and lay him on his side in his crib so that you have access to his back (if the baby is old enough to sleep on his stomach, then you can lay him that way instead).
3. Pat the baby on the back slowly and rhythmically while making a shushing sound just over his ear (not directly into it). The shushing is meant to emulate the sounds that the baby was exposed to in the womb.
4. If the baby starts crying and is inconsolable with the shushing and patting, pick him up and continue the shushing and patting.
5. When he calms down completely, lay him back down in the crib and continue the shushing and patting for a few minutes until he starts to become sleepy, then slow down the process.
6. Don't stop touching him and shushing him until he's deeply asleep.
7. Once you've done this for several days or weeks, your baby will get used to falling asleep faster and faster without being picked up and eventually will not need your support at all.

There are a number of reasons to recommend these more gentle approaches to sleep training. First, many parents report experiencing less emotional distress, and less guilt in particular, when implementing these methods as compared to the extinction methods. Second, for parents with a great deal of patience and support, these methods do prove to be effective. Third, the more gentle methods are more likely to be consistently implemented because they cause less distress for the whole family. This consistency, again, may be one of the most important factors responsible for successful sleep training. Here's what one parent had to say about the advantages of no-cry methods:

JENNA'S STORY

The No-Cry Nights

I loved Pantley's *No-Cry Sleep Solution* recommendations— we used different forms of her methods on a number of occasions, using the "gentle removal plan" to get her from nursing back down to rocking back down to patting back down to putting herself back to sleep. Starting when she was about 11 months old, we would comfort her without picking her up, and leave. If she cried, we went back in, picked her up until she was calm, and then left again. It took a few nights of some serious work at bedtime, but by the sixth night, she wasn't waking in the middle of the night anymore. I can't tell you the difference it made for everyone in our family to sleep all night. The whole family was healthier, happier, and more patient and loving.

As with any approach, there are also some points against this set of gentler methods. First, almost all the sleep experts agree that these methods require a lot more time, commitment, and patience on the part of the parent than the "quicker fixes" of extinction or gradual extinction. As a result, severely sleep-deprived parents may give up too soon to get the promised results. Second, these methods often require a great deal of the mother's own loving attention and time—resources that the mother may be sorely lacking by the time she has decided to sleep train her child. The father, although encouraged to participate in some of these approaches, is regarded as more of a support figure. Finally, a great number of parents report that many of these methods end up *encouraging* dependence on the parent during bedtime and naps, rather than discouraging it. Because the parent is required to be present during sleep transitions, albeit less so over days and weeks, some children begin to feel more frustration, rather than less, at their mother's unwillingness to soothe them in a consistent manner. One mother put it this way:

CHRISTINE'S STORY
Absence Makes the Child Sleep Longer

I tried all of the no-cry, pick-up-put-down, pat-his-back stuff, and none of it worked for us. It just escalated the problems, actually. When Lucas was 9 months old, he would take one look at me inching my hand away from his crib and start wailing. It got to the point that even a slight sigh or shift in my chair got him hollering, because he knew in the next minute I would move my chair just a little bit away. I was spending more time (up to 2 hours) getting him to go back to sleep without nursing than he would actually stay asleep (like, 40 minutes). Then I'd have to haul my butt out of bed to start the whole routine over again. I finally gave up and decided that I was a total idiot, since all I needed to do was nurse him for 10 minutes and we could all go back to sleep for another 3 to 4 hours. Not ideal but an improvement over some of those "hush-hush programs" we tried.

No Matter What Method You Choose . . .

Simply listing the top sleep-training methods would not be useful to most parents. Which one's the best? What will work most effectively for your child? We can't answer these questions for you because we firmly believe that the answer is *it depends*. It depends on your own childhood experiences of being parented, your parenting philosophies, your particular child's personality, your culture, your family structure (single or with a partner, other kids or not, grandparents in or out of the picture), your employment situation, and your childcare arrangements. What we have emphasized throughout the book is how important developmental timing is in the implementation of whatever method you choose. Though we won't point you toward any specific approach, here are some guidelines gleaned from our professional and very personal experiences with sleep-training methods:

- Pick the approach that feels right for you. That means go with a sleep-training method that seems to match your parenting philosophy or approach in general. And try to ignore the naysayers—whether they're the (lying) mothers at the park whose babies slept through the night at 8 weeks;

Grandma, who thinks you're spoiling your child by nursing her to sleep; or the nanny who eyes you with suspicion when you let your baby so much as whimper before naptime. You know your child best, and ultimately, you have to live with your parenting choices.

- Pick a method that seems to address your child's personality. We briefly reviewed some temperamental styles and their implications for sleep training, but our treatment was necessarily superficial. Trust your gut on this one. For example, if you have a particularly sensitive child who cannot tolerate being separated from you no matter what, then straight cry-it-out may be soul-destroying for you and just plain ineffective for your child.

- Pick the approach you know you can stick with and give it a fair try. That means apply the method consistently, and do so for at least a week.

- Related to the previous point, keep in mind that things often get worse before they get better. Children already have sleep habits by the time we decide to sleep train them. Breaking those habits may involve some disruption and disorganization, and even outright rebellion, on the part of your baby or toddler. As a result your child may sleep less or wake more frequently before she settles into a new routine.

- If one method doesn't work for your baby (or your family as a whole), then pick something else. Keep your mind as open as possible to different strategies and try to opt out of the polarizing "mommy wars." There is no method that makes you an intrinsically more "sensitive" parent, no matter what the sleep experts tell you.

- Whatever sleep-training method you choose, develop a concrete plan *during the daytime hours*, when you feel maximally rested. Do *not* come up with a strategy in the throes of the fifth waking of the night, at 4 a.m. Sleep deprivation and inevitable frustration will make this middle-of-the-night plan less feasible and more irrational, and its implementation more haphazard. We suspect that many a marriage has been sorely tested in the wee hours by the eruption of sleep-training debates.

- Find yourself a person to support you through the sleep-training process. Ideally, this someone should not be your partner, who likely is feeling the same level of stress you are. Find a colleague who's gone through the process, or a family member who can cheer you on, or a friend who can take you out for a meal during the worst of it. There are also some fantastic "mommy" support groups on the Internet that can serve as powerful cheering squads.

6

Sleep Setbacks and How to Handle Them

SO LET'S SAY THAT YOU HAVE FOUND the most appropriate sleep-training method to suit your and your child's needs, you have followed all the sage advice from your chosen sleep-training gurus, and you've applied this method at precisely the right developmental window. Your child is now sleeping beautifully through the night and is taking regular naps for reasonable durations. He is a bright, bubbly, joyful child who is a delight to be with most of the time. You, in turn, are also sleeping glorious long stretches of time. You are finally feeling sane. You can think better, your mood is brighter, your appetite has returned, your depression has lifted, you have begun to socialize again with friends. You finally can enjoy your child or children and start living the happy family life you once imagined.

And then, *bam*! One day your perfect sleeper goes from sleeping 12 hours through the night to waking up every hour and a half. She's screaming again, crying for something, waking up and unable to fall back to sleep. She is suddenly refusing to nap. The same routines are no longer working to calm her. The same music isn't soothing anymore, the same bounce loses its hypnotic impact, the same bedtime story is slapped out of your hand in toddler disgust. Maybe it's just a bad day or night? No, it goes on for days and sometimes weeks. Your sanity now feels very much at risk.

We've heard this account from many parents and have experienced it firsthand. It's called a sleep setback. Sleep setbacks are relatively predictable, and your own mother or grandmother may have told you about similar experiences with her children. Often these setbacks are referred to as *sleep regressions*. We are not terribly fond of this phrase because *regression* implies a return to old patterns, old habits, more infantile forms of behavior. And in fact we believe that these "regressions" are often leaps forward, not backward—corresponding to a shift in the child's stage of cognitive and emotional development. However, to parents, they can definitely *feel* like regressions. After finally getting yourself a stretch of 6, 8, or even more hours of sleep per night, going back to 1- or 2-hour bursts of it feels like a diabolical form of torture. For the parent, it *does* feel like the child has reverted back to patterns from early infancy when she was waking every hour or two to be fed, soothed, rocked, or cajoled back to sleep. But by now, most parents no longer have the support of friends and family who were there to commiserate when the baby was brought home from the hospital. By now, some parents have perhaps joyfully announced, maybe even boasted, about their child's hard-won sleep skills. And suddenly, overnight, with seemingly no rhyme or reason, all those skills have vanished. What's happened to your perfect little sleeper?

Sensitive Windows of Development

There are a number of reasons why your child seems to have lost his sleep skills. We mention a number of them in the next section, but perhaps the most common explanation is that your child has matured and entered one of the sensitive, vulnerable stages outlined in Chapter 4. These are the stages that were difficult for sleep training to begin with. As we discussed in detail in the second and third chapters, these periods are created by cognitive advances and the emotional challenges they engender, and they are particularly troublesome periods for teaching an infant or toddler to sleep on his own. In the same way, entry into these stages may cause the psychological upheavals your child is going through now, and these may be responsible for sleep disruptions when none were present before. So, if your child's age places him in one of the "sensitive windows" outlined in Figure 3 on pages 130 to 131, this could explain why you are experiencing these difficulties now.

So what do you do about these major sleep disruptions, and how do you reteach your child to sleep on her own? The answer to the first part of this question is perhaps difficult to swallow, but it is the best advice we have: wait. Wait until the sensitive period is over. Do minimize the damage by keeping to the same sleep routines you have already established. Also, try several booster sessions of the sleep-training method you originally applied. Try to be consistent with sleep routines while at the same time providing as much emotional support as you can muster, and recognize that the developmental issues you are coping with now are not the same as those you weathered when you first initiated sleep training. But aside from this, waiting this phase out is probably the most realistic option. Something about the current developmental window has set off an allergic reaction to sleep habits already formed, and whatever it is likely will continue to obstruct your efforts. This sensitive window will pass. And once it does, your child will probably start sleeping well again, with or without additional intervention from you. If there haven't been any major biological or psychological traumas, we can pretty much guarantee that she will come through this stage unscathed and revert back to being a champion sleeper, with the skills and confidence she initially gained through sleep training. And as you might predict by now, we highly recommend that you wait until the end of this sensitive stage before attempting any new sleep-training program. We hope that just knowing how "normal" these setbacks are, and knowing that they are likely to be temporary, will help you through this stage.

In the meantime, while you're waiting for this transition period to end, take care of yourself. Take long walks, treat yourself to trashy novels, or demand daily back rubs from your partner. Take special care of yourself *and* your partner. Figure out a system that provides you with additional hours of sleep to get through this stressful period. Hire a babysitter once in a while. Get anyone else to take care of your child or children for a few hours during the day so that you can nap yourself and be in top form to weather this challenging time. As much as these sensitive stages are difficult, they are also times of delightful and exciting changes: the dawning of joint attention and that first sense of interpersonal togetherness at 8 to 11 months, the advent of language and social understanding at 17 to 21 months, and so forth. If you are able to eke out enough sleep to keep relatively sane, then you will better appreciate and enjoy the leaps and bounds by which your child is becoming a real little person. For us, what maintained our sanity during these challenging periods was the knowledge that each onslaught of changes was normal, predictable, wondrous, and *not forever.*

Other Common Causes of Sleep Disruptions

In addition to the pendulum swings of stage transitions, there are a number of common childhood issues that disrupt healthy sleep habits. The first is teething. There is a fascinating amount of variation among babies in terms of how much pain they experience during teething episodes. Some pediatricians have had the gall to suggest to us that teething doesn't actually cause pain—it just "seems" like that to us. Most parents, however, have had the heartbreaking feeling of watching a child wail through a teething episode, rubbing his gums like mad and biting on anything that passes his way. Teething can disrupt sleep for the obvious reason: pain is difficult to sleep through. But teething is also often accompanied by a runny nose, fever, congestion, coughing from all the drool that gets stuck in the back of the throat, and rashes around the mouth or anal area—all difficult symptoms to fall asleep and stay asleep with! Teething episodes can last for as little as a day or as long as many weeks. Diagnosing the problem can be critical for your sanity and, importantly, for helping your child by providing pain relief and emotional support.

Another common cause for sleep disruptions is sickness (anything from the common colds that are weekly plagues for us in winter to more serious illnesses). Traveling and having guests visit your home can also be enormously disruptive for babies' and toddlers' sleep schedules.

All of these circumstances—teething, illness, traveling—require parents to respond to their children's difficulties falling and staying asleep with sensitivity and more persistent soothing strategies. So, most parents will cuddle, rock, nurse, and otherwise comfort their children for as long as it takes to relieve their pain and anxieties during stressful times. Of course! But the problem is that by the time the causes for these sleep disruptions disappear, those hard-won sleep skills too may have dissolved.

Context Matters

One reason sleep training usually is not a one-shot deal for families is that as the child develops, the world around her also changes. This important aspect of sleep training has received little attention in our book so far. The issue is not specific to learning how to go to sleep on one's own: it is a fundamental aspect of all kinds of learning, especially in the early years of life but also, to some degree, throughout the lifespan. It's the role of context. When we learn a new skill, we use all the cognitive resources at our disposal, and it seems as though these cognitive powers alone either permit learning to occur or are found insufficient to the task. But learning relies on much more than what's going on inside our heads. It also relies on what's going on in the environment.

When a child learns to count, he does indeed require a brain that's mature enough to grasp the way numbers stand for a sequence of objects. He needs the language skills to utter words that stand for numerical placement. He also needs joint attention and social referencing so that he can pay attention to what is being taught by his parent or teacher. These are all the requirements for counting that rest within the child. But he needs a great deal from outside his skin. He needs a parent or teacher patient enough to repeat numbers while pointing to objects. He needs a set of objects that are the right size and shape, that are lined up in such a way as to highlight their "countability." He also needs to be well fed and well rested so that he can concentrate on the task at hand. And he needs a well-lit room and a learning space where the objects to be counted stand out from their background and are available to be pointed to or manipulated. Learning depends on context.

We take this for granted and intuitively prepare contexts to help children learn whatever it is we're trying to teach them. We don't try to teach a child the names for colors in a dark room, and we don't try to teach table manners to a child who has the flu, or who is extremely hungry, or who wants nothing more than to be finished eating and go out to play. We adapt the context to the task and the task to the context. And the child's learning depends on the context in which he's taught. Finally, skills that are not yet completely formed, or that are easily lost or forgotten, are best maintained when we reproduce the context in which they were learned. Table manners take a long time to perfect, but if we want to keep them from vanishing, we practice them again and again in a calm context that helps children focus (for example, in a high chair) with patient family members who eat alongside them.

The role of context in learning and maintaining optimal sleep habits could not be more critical. We don't teach children to sleep on their own when they're overtired, or going to sleep at Grandma's house, or when their stuffed animal is AWOL. And we make sure that the lights are dim, the room warm, and the belly full. We intuitively understand the importance of comfort and consistency, and we carefully prepare the child's environment to maximize the chances of successful sleep training. Then, once sleep training has begun to "take," we set up bedtime practices that will ensure its continued success. We wait until the child is tired, but not overtired, we calm her down with stories and other peaceful activities, we sing familiar songs, ones that before long will become bedrock routine, we set the lights at just the correct dimness, and we make sure that every nuance of our own behavior conforms to our child's expectations. That's what gives sleep habits the best chance of setting, like a plaster cast, and becoming more solid over time.

So one of the most common causes of sleep setbacks is, simply, a change in the context of going to sleep—often a change that we're unaware of, or that we don't see as important, and sometimes a change that we can't control. Changes in context come in all varieties. Some are obvious, like a change in location. Sleep habits have a tendency to go out the window when you're on vacation, or sleeping in a hotel room or a relative's guest room. This is one reason why family "vacations" may not be so restful during the early years. Other obvious changes in context may be the other people involved. If Mom is always present when baby goes to sleep, then her absence can have a formidable impact on sleep habits, and Dad may be at an utter loss while Mom is whooping it up with her girlfriend in Mazatlán. But these changes are usually temporary, and avoidable.

Other changes in context are not so easy to remedy. When winter turns to spring and spring to summer, your baby may have to get used to going to sleep with light pouring through the curtains. And even the smallest sliver of light may be enough to change her fundamental sense that it's not bedtime yet. When a new baby comes along, a new sibling, this can also cause a major upheaval for your previously perfect sleeper. Now you're different in so many ways. You don't read as many books at bedtime. You're tired, you're less patient, you smell funny (it's all that fresh spit-up on your sweatshirt) and so forth. And there are different noises in the house. Things aren't as quiet as they used to be. Such changes are hard to ameliorate, and they may have drastic effects on your child's sleep habits. Previously champion sleepers may suddenly take to lying awake, chanting or whining, or rattling the bars of their cribs like little criminals. All because the context of going to sleep has changed in some pivotal way.

The solution for sleep setbacks caused by changes such as these is obvious: change the context back to whatever worked best or whatever was in place until now. If you can. Of course, if it's a change in season, from winter to spring, you won't have much luck changing it back for another half year or so. But you can, instead, install heavy curtains to block out the light coming through the window. Often the best you can do is to approximate the former context. If the noise level in the house is the problem, put a white-noise generator, or even a simple fan, next to the baby's crib. The trick to finding the right solution is pinpointing what's different. Often some detective work is required. Whatever has changed in the lighting, atmosphere, sound level, or *you* may not be obvious, even though it is sufficiently potent to affect your child's sleep. Babies and toddlers are exquisitely sensitive little beings, and their nervous systems are tuned to many perceptual aspects of their environment that completely escape your attention. And they *like* familiarity. So, if a sleep setback seems to have no other cause, try to imagine yourself in that crib. Tune your eyes, ears, nose, and skin to your baby's world, and you'll probably figure out the problem.

•

We hope that this chapter and this book on the whole have given you some bottom-line solutions for resolving your child's sleep problems, whether they've arisen for the first time or after many months of blissful snoring. And we trust that these pages have given you a deeper appreciation for how your baby sees, feels, and thinks about the world, even if those insights don't always translate neatly into words. Parenting is, after all, a highly intuitive process. But if you can support your instincts with a real understanding of how your child's cognitive and emotional development progresses, your intuition will be sharper and more seasoned than before. And you'll be able to change your child's sleep patterns with clarity of mind and confidence.

You're the expert now. Good luck with the job ahead.

Acknowledgments

We'd like to thank members of the publishing team at HarperCollins Canada for their support and guidance regarding the first edition of this book. To Brad Wilson, our thanks for helping us through the jungle of choices about editorial structure as well as design issues. Brad has been encouraging about the project from the start. Noelle Zitzer had many good ideas to help guide our thinking about the tone and style of the manuscript. Thanks also to Noelle for the catchy subtitles throughout the volume. And to Rob Firing, thanks for some novel ideas (and questionable jokes) about all phases of the work.

We'd also like to acknowledge Matthew Lore and his team at The Experiment; we are very grateful for the enthusiasm and care they have given us through preparations for this U.S. edition of our book.

We'd also like to thank the many parents (mostly mothers) who have contributed to the book with their personal stories and very quotable accounts of agonies and ecstasies during the great sleep wars.

Thanks to Ruben and Julian for being model children and letting us think we really did know a thing or two about developmental timing. You were the inspiration for this book in more ways than two. Our sincere thanks go to Flo and Marc Granic,

Isabel's parents, for helping to pay some of the bills so our stress could be harnessed toward productivity rather than just getting through the day alive. To Marc, thanks as well for retracting your skepticism where this book was concerned. You believed that we could do it, and we did. To Flo, thank you for coming over countless times to look after our boys, to look after Isabel when she needed it, and to help both of us catch up on critical hours of sleep—sleep without which this book would have never been written. Thanks also to Allan and Roz for their enormous enthusiasm for our writing.

And finally, this book came to fruition after listening to friends, neighbors, and each other complaining endlessly about the challenges of getting through the night with our babies or toddlers. Thanks to all of you for continuing to complain until we came up with solutions.

Bibliography

Bakeman, Roger, L. B. Adamson, M. Konner, and R. G. Barr. "Sequential
  Analyses of !Kung Infant Communication: Inducing and Recruiting." In
  Change and Development: Issues of Theory, Method, and Application,
  edited by Eric Amsel and K. Ann Renninger, 173–192. Mahwah, NJ:
  Lawrence Erlbaum Associates, 1997.

Campos, J. J., D. I. Anderson, M. A. Barbu-Roth, E. M. Hubbard, M. J.
  Hertenstein, and D. Witherington. "Travel Broadens the Mind." *Infancy* 1
  (2000): 149–219.

Case, Robbie. *Intellectual Development: Birth to Adulthood.* New York:
  Academic Press, 1985.

Case, Robbie. "The Whole Child: Toward an Integrated View of Young
  Children's Cognitive, Social, and Emotional Development." In *Psychological
  Bases for Early Education,* edited by A. D. Pellegrini, 155–184. New York:
  Wiley, 1988.

Case, Robbie, Y. Okamoto, S. Griffin, A. McKeough, C. Bleiker, B. Henderson,
  and K. M. Stephenson. "The Role of Central Conceptual Structures in
  the Development of Children's Thought." *Monographs of the Society for
  Research in Child Development* 61 (1996): Serial No. 246.

Chess, Stella, and Alexander Thomas. *Temperament: Theory and Practice.*
  New York: Brunner/Mazel, 1996.

Dunn, Judy. *The Beginnings of Social Understanding.* Cambridge, MA:
  Harvard University Press, 1988.

Ferber, Richard. *Solve Your Child's Sleep Problems.* New York: Fireside, 2006.

Friday, Nancy. *Jealousy.* New York: Perigord, 1985.

Hogg, Tracy, with Melinda Blau. *Secrets of the Baby Whisperer: How to Calm,
  Connect, and Communicate with Your Baby.* New York: Ballantine, 2001.

Izard, Carroll E. "Emotion–Cognition Relationships and Human Development."
  In *Emotions, Cognition, and Behavior,* edited by Carroll E. Izard, Jerome

Kagan, and Robert B. Zajonc, 17–37. Cambridge, MA: Cambridge University Press, 1984.

Kagan, Jerome. *Galen's Prophecy: Temperament in Human Nature.* New York: Basic Books, 1994.

Kramer, Peter D. *Listening to Prozac.* New York: Penguin, 1994.

Mahler, Margaret S., Fred Pine, and Anni Bergman. *The Psychological Birth of the Human Infant.* New York: Basic Books, 1975.

Mindell, Jodi A., B. Kuhn, D. S. Lewin, L. J. Meltzer, and A. Sadeh. "Behavioral Treatment of Bedtime Problems and Night Wakings in Infants and Young Children." *Sleep* 29 (2006): 1263–1276.

Pascual-Leone, Juan, and Doba Goodman. "Intelligence and Experience: A Neopiagetian Approach." *Instructional Science* 8 (1979): 301–367.

Piaget, Jean. *The Origins of Intelligence in Children.* New York: International Universities Press, 1952.

Sander, L. W. "Infant and Caretaking Environment: Investigation and Conceptualization of Adaptive Behavior in a System of Increasing Complexity." In *Explorations in Child Psychiatry*, edited by E. J. Anthony, 129–166. New York: Plenum, 1975.

Sroufe, L. Alan. *Emotional Development: The Organization of Emotional Life in the Early Years*. New York: Cambridge University Press, 1995.

Stern, Daniel N. *The First Relationship: Infant and Mother.* Cambridge, MA: Harvard University Press, 1977.

Stern, Daniel N. *The Interpersonal World of the Infant: A View from Psychoanalysis and Developmental Psychology.* New York: Basic Books, 1985.

Tomasello, Michael. "Joint Attention as Social Cognition." In *Joint Attention: Its Origins and Role in Development,* edited by Chris Moore and Philip J. Dunham, 103–130. Hillsdale, NJ: Erlbaum, 1995.

Trevarthen, Colwyn. "The Foundations of Intersubjectivity: Development of Interpersonal and Cooperative Understanding in Infants." In *The Social Foundations of Language and Thought: Essays in Honor of Jerome S. Bruner,* edited by David R. Olson, 316–342. New York: W.W. Norton & Co., 1980.

Tronick, Ed. *The Neurobehavioral and Social Emotional Development of Infants and Children.* New York: W.W. Norton & Co., 2007.

Weissbluth, Marc. *Healthy Sleep Habits, Happy Child: A Step-by-Step Program for a Good Night's Sleep.* New York: Ballantine, 2005.

Index

actions, coordination of, 22–23, 24–25, 28–31

Actions & Outcomes stage, 26, 28–31, 66–74
  sleep training during, 141–51

affection
  sensitivity to loss of, 104
  withdrawal of, 92

anxious or inhibited babies, 121, 122–23, 170

AskMoxie.com, 200–201

"attachment"-oriented sleep strategies, 202

attention
  competition for, 102–3
  focusing of, 24–25
  interpersonal, 63–66
  joint, 80–83, 85
  role in emotional stability, 50–53
  shifting of, 29–30, 33, 35
  toddler's "addiction" to, 94–95, 169

autonomy
  and competing goals, 91–93
  during Family Membership stage, 110–11
  during Interpersonal Expectancy stage, 67–71
  during Motor Initiative stage, 71–74, 146–48
  during Motor Practice stage, 83–87
  importance to sleep training, 31, 35
  locomotion and, 84, 86

babysitters, 105, 214
  during sleep training, 123

The Baby Whisperer Solves All Your Problems (Hogg), 203–4

bad dreams, 117

Baetz, Carla, 115

Barr, Ronald, 58

Basic Regulation stage, 55–62, 130
  sleep training during, 132–35

bedtime rituals, 187–88

as aid to sleep training, 160–61, 171, 174–75, 186
  and sleep training, 111

brain, growth and maturation, 15–18

Campos, Joseph, 79

Case, Robbie, 19–21, 22, 25, 35

cerebral cortex, 15–18

Chess, Stella, 120

clicking. *See* Social Referencing stage

clinginess. *See* separation distress

cognitive development, 15–47
  individual differences, 41–42
  relationship to emotional development, 19, 49–55, 98–99
  stages, 19–20, 26–27 (*see also under specific stages*)
  timetable, 18–20, 23–24
  transition between stages, 22–23, 25–28

cognitive entities, coordination of, 22–23, 24–25, 28–32

compulsive behavior, 117

context
  dependence of emotional response on, 53
  importance to sleep training, 216–20

cooperation, 90–91, 100, 109, 111–12, 120

coping responses, 51–52, 98–99

co-sleeping, 201, 202

crawling
  and increased autonomy, 84
  and social referencing, 78–79

crying
  inexplicable, 59–60, 137–38
  responding quickly to, 202

cry-it-out methods, 152, 166–67, 187–92, 202
  contrasted with Ferberizing, 196

day-night differentiation, 61–62, 132, 133–34

deception, 45
depression
    in mothers, 50–51
    and sleep deprivation, 5
"difficult" temperament, 120, 121–22
dim lighting, 203, 204, 218
disengagement, as coping response, 51–52
distraction, appearance of, 30
distress
    causes and coping responses, 50–54
    separation (*see* separation distress)
Dunn, Judy, 100

"easy" temperament, 120, 123–24, 183
emotional development, 49–124
    individual differences, 106–8, 117–25,
        173–74
    relationship to cognitive development,
        19, 49–55, 98–99
    and sleep setbacks, 213–15
    stages, 55–117, 130–31
    stages poorly suited to sleep training,
        55–62, 66–71, 74–83, 87–96, 100–106,
        111–17, 130–31, 132–35, 141–45,
        151–58, 162–68, 172–75, 180–83,
        213–15
    stages well suited to sleep training,
        63–66, 71–74, 83–87, 97–100, 106–11,
        130–31, 135–41, 145–51, 158–62,
        168–72, 176–79
emotional displacement, 53
emotional stability, importance to sleep
    training, 30–31
emotions
    control over, 51–53, 101–2, 108–9, 174
    dependence on context, 53
empathy, 45
environment
    effect on cognitive development, 42
    effect on sleep training, 216–20
    effect on temperament, 119
events
    ability to anticipate, 36–37, 64–66,
        67–68
    thinking about, 35–36
experience
    adapting to, 120–21
    effect on development of cerebral
        cortex, 16–18
    effect on temperament, 119

"extinction." *See* cry-it-out methods;
    gradual extinction

false-belief understanding, 42–45, 112–17,
    180–81
family membership, sense of, 86, 93–94
Family Membership stage, 106–11, 131
    sleep training during, 176–79
feedings, 58–59, 61, 140, 150–51, 168, 193
Ferber, Richard, 189, 192–98
Ferberizing, 189, 192–98
    contrasted with cry-it-out methods,
        196
    and working memory, 198
Friday, Nancy, 103
frontal cortex, 22

game-playing
    coordination of social roles through,
        37–38
    expectation of parents' response to, 70
    increased intricacy of, 73
    initiation by baby, 67–68, 70
    socio-dramatic, 110, 178–79
gaze
    averting, 51–52
    avoiding, 70
    reciprocal, 63–64, 66
goals
    acting toward, 28–29
    competing, 38, 91–93, 165–66
    expression of, 36–37
    manipulation of others, 101–2
    modification of, 92–93
    relationship to rules, 40, 100–101
    sharing of, 75–76, 85–86, 88–90, 109
    understanding of others', 38–39, 80–81
gradual extinction, 192–98, 203

Healthy Sleep Habits, Healthy Child
    (Weissbluth), 189, 199–201
Hogg, Tracy, 203–4
Honing Skills stage, 27, 34–35, 83–87
    sleep training during, 158–62
*How to Solve Your Child's Sleep
    Problems* (Ferber), 196–97

illness, sleep setbacks caused by, 216
impulse control, 98–99, 109
independence. *See* autonomy

individual variations, in rates of
  development, 41–42, 106–8, 117–24
infant initiative, period of, 71–74
"intermittent" reinforcement, of habits, 195–96
Interpersonal Attention stage, 63–66, 130
  sleep training during, 135–41
interpersonal confusion, 134
Interpersonal Expectancy stage, 66–71, 130
  sleep training during, 141–45
interrelational stage, 20, 35–47, 91–117,
  162–83
intersubjectivity, 63–66

jealousy, 41, 102–5, 173–75
joint attention, 80–83
  as prerequisite for language use, 85, 88–90
  and separation distress, 156–58

Kagan, Jerome, 10–11, 120–21
Kramer, David, 104

language
  and autonomy, 110–11
  naming explosion, 36–37, 88
  relationship to joint attention, 85–86,
    159–60
  stringing together of words, 35–37, 88,
    97–100
  use of single words, 34–35
"late practicing" phase, 84
lying, 45

"magico-phenomenalistic causality," 142.
  See also Actions & Outcomes stage;
  Interpersonal Expectancy stage
Mahler, Margaret, 66–67, 72, 84
McCall, Robert B., 107
McKenna, James J., 201
mental states, 44–45
Mindell, Jodi, 189
"mommy wars," 4, 208–9
mood, effect of sleep deprivation on, 5–7
moral development, 40
mother
  coordination with, 58–60
  eye contact with, 18
  reciprocity with infant, 63–66
Motherese (infant-directed vocalizing),
  63–64
motor actions

coordination of, 22–23, 24–25, 28–32,
  55–62
mastery of, 30–31, 34–35
Motor Initiative stage, 71–74, 130
  sleep training during, 145–51
Motor Practice stage, 83–87, 130
  sleep training during, 158–62

naming explosion, 36–37, 88
naps, during the day, 6, 199, 200–201
night terrors, 117
Nighttime Parenting (Sears), 201
no-cry methods of sleep training, 201–7
The No-Cry Sleep Solution (Pantley),
  201, 205
nonverbal cues, 78–79, 81
nursing
  baby to sleep, 187–88, 203
  time between feedings, 58–59, 61, 140,
    150–51

objectivity, 43
objects
  grabbing and sucking on, 18, 30
  reaching for while tracking, 28–29
  searching for vanished, 18–19, 32, 73,
    77, 153–55
  tracking of moving, 24
  use of in coping with loneliness, 110–11
Orienting stage, 24–29, 55–66
  sleep training during, 132–41
ownership, 38–39, 93

Pantley, Elizabeth, 201, 202–3, 205
parents
  attention and emotional stability, 50–53
  attentiveness to, 81–83
  coordination with, 58–60, 63–64
  deciding when to begin, 136–41
  differentiation from, 66–71
  feelings of guilt about sleep training, 3–4,
    152–53, 166–67, 189, 191, 204–5, 208–9
  need to take care of selves, 139, 214
  nonverbal cues, 78–79, 81, 134
  toddler's "addiction" to attention from,
    94–95
  withdrawal of affection by, 92
Pascual-Leone, Juan, 21
Perspective-Taking stage, 27, 41–47,
  111–17

physical world, fascination with, 19, 69–74, 79, 146–48, 158–62
physiology, coordination of, 55–62
Piaget, Jean, 18–20, 32, 35, 142
Point & Click stage, 26, 31–34, 73, 74–83
  sleep training during, 151–58
pointing, 32–33, 76–77, 79–80
practicing phase, 71–72
preoperational stage, 35–39
problem solving, reliance on working memory, 22

reasoning skills, 53
rebellion, 40, 52, 95, 121–22, 174
reciprocal exchange, 50, 63–69, 134
reversible actions, 34, 85
roles
  complementary, 90–91
  coordination of, 37–38
  understanding of, 86, 90–94, 102, 110, 178–79
Roles, Goals, & Language stage, 27, 35–39, 87–100
  sleep training during, 162–72
rules
  acceptance of, 108–9, 111
  understanding of, 40, 52, 100–101, 169, 171

Sander, Louis, 57–59, 71, 72
Sears, William, 201
seasons, and sleep setbacks, 219–20
self-confidence
  and ability to walk and talk, 86, 159–60
  encouraging, 182
Self-Consciousness stage, 111–17, 131
  sleep training during, 180–83
self-doubt, 89–90, 103–4
sense of family membership, 86, 93–94, 106–11
sense of self, 66–68, 89, 143
sensorimotor stage, 20, 28–35, 66–91, 132–62
separation distress, 33–34, 39, 45, 70–71, 95–96
  and babysitters, 123
  coping responses, 110
  and joint attention, 154–58
  lack of at certain stages, 64–66, 73, 100
  link to capacity to retrieve hidden objects, 77

  peaks during Social Negotiation stage, 163–65
  relationship to sense of self, 143–45
  rise of, 153–58
  "separation sensitivity," 104
  as sign it's not time to start sleep training, 138–40
  and social intelligence, 80–83
  and working memory, 64–66, 73, 146–47, 153–55
shame, 45, 103–4, 114–17, 181–82
"shush/pat" method of sleep training, 203–4
siblings
  effect on sleep training, 41
  and jealousy, 104–5
  and sleep setbacks, 219
skill dispersion, 41–42
sleep deprivation, 168
  effects of, 4–7
  inevitability of, 62, 201
  and need to start sleep training, 140–41
  and new parents, 1–3
  as obstacle to no-cry methods, 206
Sleeping Through the Night (Mindell), 189
Sleeping with Your Baby (McKenna), 201
sleep routines, and scheduling, 5, 7–8, 199–201
sleep setbacks, 211–21
  causes, 213–16
sleep training
  baby's ability to unlearn habits, 96, 135, 175, 176–77, 179, 188
  and bedtime rituals, 111, 171, 174–75
  cognitive stages poorly suited to, 33–34
  cost-benefit ratio, 138–39
  definition, 7
  during Basic Regulation stage, 62
  during Family Membership stage, 111
  during Interpersonal Attention stage, 66
  during Interpersonal Expectancy stage, 71
  during Motor Initiative stage, 74
  during Self-consciousness stage, 117
  during Social Comparison stage, 105–6
  during Social Negotiation stage, 95–96
  during Social Referencing stage, 82–83
  during Social Stabilization stage, 100
  effect of siblings, 41

emotional stages poorly suited to, 55–62, 66–71, 74–83, 87–96, 100–106, 111–17, 130–31, 132–35, 141–45, 151–58, 162–68, 172–75, 180–83, 213–15

emotional stages well suited to, 63–66, 71–74, 83–87, 97–100, 106–11, 130–31, 135–41, 145–51, 158–62, 168–72, 176–79

importance of context, 216–20

importance of emotional stability, 30–31, 45

importance of timing of, 8–12

methods, 186–209

necessity of, 4–6

parents' feelings of guilt about, 3–4, 152–53, 166–67, 189, 191, 204–5, 208–9

"sensitive windows" of development, 213–14

and temperament, 119, 121–24

when to choose a method, 209

"slow-to-warm-up" temperament, 120–21

smiling
increased frequency of, 60–61, 63
reciprocal, 50, 63, 134

social cognition, 38–39, 43, 44–45

Social Comparison stage, 100–106, 131
sleep training during, 172–75

social cues, 78–79, 81

social intelligence, 80–83, 108–9

Social Maneuvering stage, 27, 39–41, 100–111
sleep training during, 172–75

Social Negotiation stage, 87–96, 131
sleep training during, 162–68

Social Referencing stage, 33–35, 74–83, 130
and language use, 88–90
sleep training during, 151–58

social roles
coordination of, 37–38
understanding of, 86, 90–94, 102, 110, 178–79

"social smile," 60–61

Social Stabilization stage, 97–100, 131
sleep training during, 168–72

social world
becomes secondary to physical world, 69–74, 146–48
increased involvement in, 74–83

Sroufe, Alan, 49

states
coordination of, 55–62
transition between, 60

Stern, Daniel, 63–66

"still face procedure," 50–52

stranger anxiety, 82

swaddling, 149–50, 204

symbolic stage, 35–39

teething, 215

temperament, 118–24. *See also under specific styles*
and choice of sleep-training method, 208
styles, 119–21

temper tantrums, 166, 167–68, 174

Terrible Twos, 39–41, 93, 162–72

territoriality, 38–39, 93

theory of mind, 42–45, 112–13, 180–81

Thomas, Alexander, 120

Tomasello, Michael, 80–81

travel, sleep setbacks caused by, 216, 218–19

Trevarthen, Colwyn, 64

Tronick, Ed, 50–52

twins, and sleep training, 144–45, 149

2–3–4 Rule, 200–201

visual cliff, 78–79

vocalization. *See also* language
to cause parent to return, 81–82, 169
with expectation of response, 23, 33, 50–51, 67–69, 70
to express wants or needs, 85–86, 91–93
Motherese (infant-directed), 63–64

waking, frequently because of hunger, 140

walking, 84, 86

Weissbluth, Marc, 189, 199–201

white-noise generators, 151, 219, 220

working memory
as catalyst for cognitive development, 20–23, 28–29, 66
and Ferberizing, 198
and separation distress, 64–66, 73, 146, 153–55